P9-DTQ-620

SINUS SURVIVAL

SINUS SURVIVAL

A SELF-HELP GUIDE
FOR ALLERGIES, BRONCHITIS,
COLDS, AND SINUSITIS

DR. ROBERT S. IVKER

FOREWORD BY GILBERT W. LEVITT, M.D.

Jeremy P. Tarcher/Perigee

JEREMY P. TARCHER/PERIGEE BOOKS
are published by
The Putnam Publishing Group
200 Madison Avenue
New York, N.Y. 10016

Library of Congress Cataloging-in-Publication Data

Ivker, Robert S.
    Sinus survival : a self-help guide for allergies, bronchitis, colds, and sinusitis /
Robert S. Ivker.—Rev. ed.
    p.   cm.
    Includes bibliographical references.
    ISBN 0-87477-684-8
    1. Sinusitis—Popular works.   2. Cold (Disease)—Popular works.
3. Respiratory allergy—Popular works.   4. Bronchitis—Popular works.
I. Title.
RF425.I85   1991
616.2—dc20   91-34424
                                                                  CIP

Copyright © 1988, 1992 by Robert S. Ivker

All rights reserved. No part of this work may be reproduced or transmitted in any
form by any means, electronic or mechanical, including photocopying and
recording, or by any information storage or retrieval system, except as may be
expressly permitted by the 1976 Copyright Act or in writing by the publisher.
Requests for such permissions should be addressed to:

Jeremy P. Tarcher, Inc.
5858 Wilshire Blvd., Suite 200
Los Angeles, CA 90036

Published in association with Whole Health Press. Distributed by St. Martin's

Design by Mauna Eichner

Manufactured in the United States of America

To my parents,
Thelma and Morris,
whose love helped to awaken
the healer within me.

CONTENTS

ACKNOWLEDGMENTS

There are so many who have made significant contributions to *Sinus Survival*. Friends, relatives, and others who have become friends as a result of our working together on this project, you have lent your time, energy, expertise, support, and love. The outcome of our combined efforts is my first book, a creation that fills me with pride, normal sinuses, and a state of health and vitality that feels indescribably wonderful. From the bottom of my heart I thank all of you.

I would also like to thank the many patients who taught me most of what I know about sinuses, and God, for the faith, creativity, and inspiration to make it all possible.

FOREWORD

In an age of ultra-specialization and high-tech medicine it is very refreshing to find a self-help book so well grounded in basic science and common sense and so practical in its application. Dr. Ivker has written *Sinus Survival* as if he were sitting in his exam room speaking to one of his patients. The overall message is hope in a framework of practical methods of action, and this permeates every page of the book. For the sinus sufferer, enjoyment of life again becomes a possibility; for those concerned about the health hazards accompanying air pollution there is a method; for people with chronic diseases seeking a complement to traditional medicine, one is provided; and for a population confronted with the environmental air pollution inevitably leading to an epidemic of respiratory disease, the seeds to redirect our destiny are planted.

As a medical self-help book I found *Sinus Survival* to be extremely practical and amazingly helpful for both patients and physicians. I enthusiastically recommend it to my sinus-suffering patients, as well as to my medical colleagues in family practice and otolaryngology (ear, nose, and throat). The book offers a wealth of remedial options for a problem that a large number of members of the medical profession find extremely frustrating to treat. In using his own case history as a model, and with his vast experience in treating several thousand sinus sufferers, combined with his gift as a teacher and a writer, Dr. Ivker clearly describes and outlines the diagnosis and treatment of acute and chronic sinusitis. By reading this book, the sinus sufferer will feel—possibly for the first time—

both understood and in much greater control of his or her condition.

In his discussion of air pollution as a causative factor of chronic sinus disease, he takes another bold step in providing methods using today's technology to deal with this aspect of the problem.

Patients that I know have especially benefited from his holistic approach to the problem. In addition to medications and surgery, he offers the reader practical advice as to what they can do to support their own immune system and increase their own power for self-healing. One's healing process changes from that of simply taking multiple antibiotics and having repeated surgery to engaging in a life-transforming process, with the recognition of our own healing potential as an important co-factor in our well-being.

Sinus Survival has not only provided me with an excellent tool for helping my patients, but in Rob Ivker I have found a kindred spirit as well.

Gilbert W. Levitt, M.D.
Clinical Instructor
Department of Otolaryngology/Head and Neck Surgery
University of Washington School of Medicine and Dentistry

PREFACE

In my medical career I have been responsible for the care of more than 20,000 patients with sinus problems. From 1977 to 1987, I worked hard to cure my own sinus condition (more about that later) and with my patients to dispel the belief that I and they would have to live indefinitely with the unpleasantness of sinusitis—despite the fact that conventional methods for treating it were becoming increasingly less effective.

Throughout my personal ten-year odyssey, I experimented with a myriad of therapeutic modalities, innovative techniques, and folk remedies. Most of my effort was focused on medical treatments, and those that were effective are all found in this book. This approach improved my sinuses; however, it was not until my healing journey took me into the exciting new frontier of holistic medicine that I obtained a cure. I have not had a sinus infection nor any symptoms of chronic sinusitis for almost five years. Since publication of the original edition of *Sinus Survival*, I have treated even more challenging sinus patients than I had seen before. They, too, experienced remarkable results. Through working with them, I have been able to refine some of the material from that first edition.

My need to practice "sinus survival" began in 1975 with my first sinus infection. I had suffered with seasonal allergies (also called hay fever) throughout most of my childhood, but this was something very different. Over the next three years, I had several more infections and finally developed chronic sinusitis. "Normal" for me now meant a stuffy head, frequent sinus headaches, and a lot of mucus drainage down the back of my throat. I consulted an ear, nose, and throat (ENT) specialist, who told me that there was no cure and that I would have to learn to live with it. I was stunned.

This young physician, who idealistically believed in the healing power of medical science, had just been given a strong dose of reality. The specialist's prognosis was a rude reminder that although modern medicine saves many lives and performs daily miracles, doctors are able to cure only about 25 percent of the ailments they treat. Chronic sinusitis is not among that select group. Although I had hardly been handed a death sentence, sinus disease was already having a profoundly negative impact on the quality of my life.

Ironically, it was to enhance my quality of life that I had come to Denver, Colorado, from Philadelphia in 1972. I entered a family practice residency training program, where I was taught that it was part of a family doctor's responsibility to teach patients about preventive medicine; in other words, how to stay well.

During my three years as a resident at Mercy Medical Center, I felt exhilarated whenever I caught a glimpse of the magnificent Rocky Mountains on the western edge of the city. With increasing frequency, however, that vista was obstructed with what later came to be known as the brown cloud. Air pollution was quickly becoming a problem that Denver could no longer ignore.

After completing my residency, I took my family and newly developed sinus condition to the outskirts of the city, where I began a solo family practice. Being something of an amateur statistician, I kept track of the diagnoses of all of my patients. Through the mid- to late 1970s, acute sinusitis (sinus infection) was usually fourteenth or fifteenth on my list of the top twenty diagnoses. By 1982 it had become number one, and it has headed my list ever since. While compiling data from other family practices and residencies for a medical conference

I was organizing, I found that my observation correlated with those of family doctors nationwide. Sinusitis was near the top of every list of the most common ailments being treated by family physicians. In the summer of 1981, the National Center for Health Statistics reported that chronic sinusitis had overtaken arthritis as the most common chronic disease in the United States.

I asked myself, Why this sudden epidemic of sinus disease? The answer came from above (the toxic cloud hovering over the city like a suffocating blanket) and from within, invading homes and workplaces to create increasingly polluted indoor environments. There was no escape. Residents of the Mile-High City are not alone in their suffering: Almost every major urban center in the world is plagued with air pollution.

According to the Environmental Protection Agency (EPA), more than 150 million Americans—60 percent of the population—live in areas in which the air is hazardous to their health. But what is actually happening to us as a result of breathing this filthy air? That question has still not been addressed by any governmental agency. Part of my purpose in writing this book has been to offer my own theory about the devastating impact air pollution is having on human beings. In this revised edition, I have included a section on indoor air pollution, a subject the EPA is now addressing as it identifies the multitude of pollutants found in our homes and workplaces.

Although it has not yet been conclusively proven in a laboratory, the hypothesis of an air pollution–sinus disease connection will certainly withstand scientific scrutiny. A primary function of the sinuses is to filter the air we breathe. We need only look at what we are breathing to appreciate that our sinuses are, at the very least, having to work much harder than they used to. After this book was first published late in 1988, I was invited to speak to the scientists at the Air Pollution Health Effects Laboratory at the University of California at Irvine. The director of the lab, Dr. Robert F. Phalen, has said,

"There is scientific evidence relating air pollution to significant epithelial cell damage in the nasal cavity of the rat." This is solid support for the pollution–sinus disease link.

Sales of this book in bookstores and in physicians' offices have shown an interesting pattern. Sales have been highest in the cities and states the EPA has identified as having the dirtiest air: Los Angeles, Denver, New York, Ohio, Texas, Pennsylvania, Michigan, Illinois, and Tennessee. This evidence might not be scientific, but it surely scores some circumstantial points in support of my theory.

Sinus disease is difficult to identify for both doctor and patient. Most people with a sinus infection believe they have "a cold that just won't quit." In this book I offer a clinical description of both acute and chronic sinusitis.

Using this book, you will be able to diagnose, treat, prevent, and—if you choose to make that level of commitment—cure yourself of the affliction of sinus disease. This is a condition that easily lends itself to self-healing. Those free of sinus problems will learn the potential hazards of breathing polluted air and what they can do to protect themselves through the practice of preventive medicine. *Sinus Survival* provides a practical plan for living a full and healthy lifestyle in an increasingly unhealthy environment.

This book offers you many avenues of possible relief from sinus disease. They all work. In Part I you will find many treatment options that offer rapid improvement of symptoms. Part II deals with causes and helps you to take increased responsibility not only for the condition of your sinuses but also for your overall state of health. The holistic methods described in Part II take longer to implement and they require more effort, but the improvement in your sinuses and general health will be far greater. Start with Part I, and if you are happy with the results, move on to Part II. The holistic program is a personalized approach to health based on learning to love yourself in all of the components of your life—physical, mental, emotional, spiritual, and social. Loving yourself is not a selfish indulgence, but rather a discovery, an appreciation, and an acceptance of the unique individual that you are. Through this work you will learn what feels good to you, how to provide it for yourself, and how to give more to others. You will experience a greater degree of health and vitality than you have ever had before.

PART I

AN INTRODUCTION TO SINUS DISEASE

1 WHAT ARE SINUSES?

Most people probably assume that the word *sinus* means "nose." They would be close, both anatomically and physiologically, but although the nose and sinuses are connected, they are separate parts of the body. The sinuses are air-filled cavities located behind and around the nose and eyes. In anatomy texts they are called air sinuses or paranasal sinuses. There are usually four sets, roughly divided in half for each side of the head. The halves can be asymmetrical in size and shape.

The sinuses are identified as frontal, maxillary, sphenoid, and ethmoid (Figure 1). The frontal sinuses lie above the eyes, just above the nose and behind the forehead. The maxillaries, the largest of the sinuses, are pyramid-shaped cavities located inside each cheekbone. The ethmoids, multicompartmental sinuses behind the maxillaries and between the bony orbits of the eyes, are complex labyrinths of small air pockets. The sphenoids are situated deep in the skull behind the nose, slightly below the ethmoids. The ethmoidal, sphenoidal, and maxillary sinuses are all present at birth, although the latter do not reach full development until a person is sixteen to twenty-one years of age. The frontal sinuses are not present until the age of eight.

To make mucus drainage and air exchange possible, each sinus is connected to the nasal passage by a thin duct about the size of pencil lead. The openings of the ducts are called ostia,

3

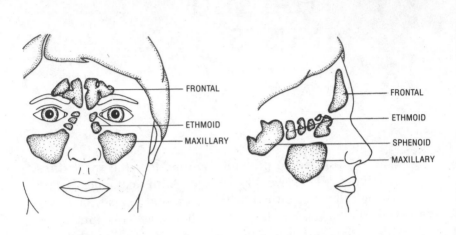

FIGURE 1   *Location of Sinuses*

and they average about two millimeters in diameter. The ducts of the maxillaries are located at the top of the sinus, making drainage difficult and blockage easy. A series of small ducts in the nasal wall drain the ethmoid sinuses; these openings are also easily blocked. Although most of the human body seems to have been created perfectly, the maxillary sinuses are a distinct exception. They appear to be better suited to four-legged animals, particularly with regard to the position of the ostia. As upright posture evolved, ease of sinus drainage diminished.

One kind of tissue, the respiratory epithelium, lines the sinuses, the nose, and the lungs. All three are part of the respiratory tract (Figure 2), which performs the essential function of breathing. The outermost part of the epithelium is called the mucosa. This is a continuous mucous membrane lining the sinuses, ducts, and nasal passages. Therefore, anything that causes a swelling in the nose can similarly affect the sinuses. On the surface of this membrane are cilia, microscopic hairlike

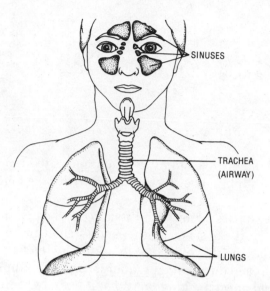

FIGURE 2   *The Respiratory Tract*

filaments that maintain a constant sweeping motion to remove the watery discharge called mucus (Figure 3).

The mucous membrane and its cilia provide a good defensive mechanism against infections. The entire mucus covering of the maxillary sinus, for example, is normally cleared every ten minutes. The mucous membrane lining the respiratory tract produces between a pint and a quart of mucus daily. The mucus traps particles that enter the nasal passage, and the cilia sweep them toward the back of the nose, after which they are swallowed and broken down by stomach acids.

No one has definitively established the exact function of the sinuses, although there is agreement that they lighten the weight of the skull. By virtue of the sinuses' location and struc-

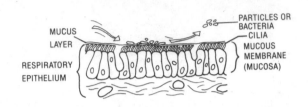

FIGURE 3   *The Sinus Lining, Healthy*

ture and the microanatomy and function of the mucous membrane, most physiologists would agree with the following conclusions.

The sinuses, along with the nose, as the upper part of the respiratory tract, serve as the body's chief protector of the lungs. They do this by acting as a *filter,* defending against viruses, dirt and dust particles, allergens, and anything airborne that would harm the lungs; as a *humidifier,* by moistening dry air that would irritate the lungs; and as a *temperature regulator,* by cooling excessively hot air and warming extremely cold air that would shock the lungs. Humans inhale about 17,000 times a day, moving the equivalent of about two gallons of air per minute. The nose and sinuses are always at work, shielding the lungs from harm. Our lungs are the vehicle through which our bodies obtain oxygen, which is vital to life itself.

The sinuses are the lungs' leading defenders against injury and illness, but their importance has been neglected by both doctors and patients. Think about a quarterback on the football field whose offensive line is weak and beginning to break down. He might not be killed, literally, but what about his health and the quality of his life? Our sinuses are being assaulted and are beginning to deteriorate. The health of our lungs, and ultimately our bodies, is at stake. Let us see how we might help preserve good health by reinforcing our first line of defense, the sinuses.

2 WHAT MAKES SINUSES SICK?

Today nearly one out of every seven Americans (34 million people) is a sinus sufferer. Sinus disease has become an epidemic. Although some factors are more critical than others, the cause of any illness is always multifaceted. The causes of this epidemic will be discussed in this chapter. They have the potential to affect adversely even the healthiest sinus. However, a person who has had previous sinus problems or whose sinuses have been weakened for any of the reasons mentioned here is already at high risk for developing sinusitis. The following agents are involved: the common cold, cigarettes and other sources of smoke, air pollution, dry air, cold air, fumes, allergies, occupational hazards, dental problems, immunodeficiency, malformations, and emotional stress.

THE COMMON COLD

The story of what has become a lifetime of sinus problems usually began with the common cold. Normally, air and mucus flow freely through the ducts connecting the nose and sinuses. Trouble starts when the system becomes obstructed, usually by a cold. The nasal mucous membrane becomes inflamed and swollen and the cold virus inactivates the cilia of the nasal membrane, causing the mucus in the nose to stagnate rather than flow (Figure 4). As a result, the mucus being produced in

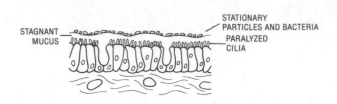

STAGNANT MUCUS

STATIONARY PARTICLES AND BACTERIA
PARALYZED CILIA

FIGURE 4 *The Sinus Lining, Sinusitis*

the sinuses cannot drain properly, and the sinuses become a breeding ground for bacteria. This pooling of stagnant mucus can easily result in a sinus infection, especially in individuals who have had previous infections.

Through the early and mid-1970s, I treated many patients who had nothing more than a bad cold. By the late seventies, and certainly by the early eighties, patients with the common cold became less frequent visitors to my office. They were being replaced by patients who greeted me with complaints such as, "Doctor, I have had this cold for the past two weeks now" (or three weeks, or several months, or in a few cases, a year or more). These people usually had sinusitis, and not until they had completed a course of antibiotics were they able to rid themselves of their "cold." It also became quite apparent that those who had never before had a sinus infection were now frequently returning with the same problem.

After a first bout with sinusitis, the mucous membrane, especially its cilia, is left in a somewhat damaged and weakened state. For many, the membrane never completely recovers, especially in an environment that is harsh on the sinuses. What I was seeing, increasingly, was that one or two "bad colds" could result in a permanently weak sinus. This impaired sinus then becomes much more susceptible to additional infections, whether from a cold or any of the other risk factors that follow.

CIGARETTES AND OTHER SOURCES OF SMOKE

Whenever a patient with a sinus infection returns to my office after completing a two-week, or longer, course of antibiotics and complains, "Doctor, I'm not any better," my first response is always a question: "Have you been smoking?" The patient often answers yes. It is extremely difficult to have healthy sinuses if you smoke cigarettes. Nicotine paralyzes the cilia. I would be hard pressed to name anything more harmful to the body's air filter than smoke of any kind. Cigarette smoke is most often involved, but cigar, pipe, campfire, and cooking smoke are also frequent villains. Marijuana and cocaine (whether smoked or snorted) are also harmful to the nasal mucous membrane.

If you are curious about what smoke does to the sinuses, take a look at the accumulation of tar and smoke particles that discolor a used cigarette filter, turning it brown or black. This will give you some idea of what is happening not only to the sinuses, but also to the lungs. At the tissue level, smoke causes irritation of the mucous membrane. The weaker the sinus, usually one that has been infected previously, the greater the level of irritation. The greater the irritation, the more inflamed the mucous membrane becomes. Inflammation of the mucous membrane results in swelling, increased mucus secretion, and damage to the cilia. This swelling may obstruct the sinuses, producing a condition very similar to that created by the common cold.

When fluids or secretions are unable to drain normally, the potential for infection is high. This principle holds true for almost any part of the human body, whether it is the bladder, bowel, lung, kidney, or middle ear space. The theory that smoking can cause sinus infections has not yet been proven. It is currently beyond the scope of science to observe what is happening to the mucous membrane in someone's sinus as it is being suffocated with smoke. However, as with the speculation on the function of the sinuses, this theory, too, has strong support among most physicians.

Those of you who are sinus sufferers but who do not smoke might not be aware that even you are not immune to the problems caused by cigarette and other types of smoke. Recent studies have shown that nonsmokers who live or work with smokers are also adversely affected. New laws that prohibit cigarette smoking in public places are helping, but we have a long way to go.

AIR POLLUTION: OUTDOOR

I was struck by a comment made several years ago by one of the Apollo astronauts. He said that the most disturbing part of his flight was seeing a grayish haze over almost every land mass on earth. What was this ugly blanket covering our beautiful planet?

Having lived in Denver, I had a good clue. The Mile-High City, one of this country's most polluted metropolitan areas, is often covered by a thick, brownish-gray pall of smog, known locally as the brown cloud. Most cities in the world are similarly afflicted, but especially those situated in valleys where temperature inversions are frequent; in cities where diesel fuel is used extensively, especially in Europe; in heavily industrialized regions; and in most areas where there are coal-fired power plants. Almost every country in the world is now familiar with this rapidly growing dilemma; it has reached such immense proportions that it is visible from space. The question is, what is this filthy air doing to the human beings who created the problem?

In Denver, the incidence of acute sinusitis has risen dramatically since the early 1970s. Since 1982, it has consistently been the most common ailment in my medical practice. Is it only a coincidence that during the same period of time air pollution has undergone a similar meteoric rise? In Denver, air pollution is most acute from mid-November to mid-January, when temperature inversions—warm air aloft trapping cold air and pollutants near the ground—are most common. This also happens to be the time of year when Denver's doctors see the greatest number of sinus infections. Many people who work in the center of the city or in other highly polluted areas are aware of the connection between their sinus congestion and sinus headaches on days with particularly bad air quality.

There is scientific evidence to implicate carbon monoxide as the most dangerous element of air pollution. Why? Because, in high enough concentrations, it is capable of killing people with weak hearts and lungs. It is also the component of air pollution most often measured, and we know that about 25 percent of it comes from vehicle emissions. But carbon monoxide is an odorless and colorless gas. What is that stuff that we can see—the brown cloud—and what is it doing to our sinuses when we breathe it?

Visible pollution consists primarily of the following elements: particulates, oxides of sulfur, oxides of nitrogen, hydrocarbons, and ozone. Particulates are tiny particles of dust, sand, cinders, soot, smoke, and liquid droplets found in the atmosphere. They come from a variety of sources, including roads, farm fields, construction sites, factories, power plants, fireplaces, wood-burning stoves, windblown dust, and diesel and car exhaust. When inhaled, larger particles (those greater than ten microns in diameter, a tenth the size of a human hair) are known to lodge in the nose and sinuses. After all, what is a filter for?

Oxides of sulfur, especially sulfur dioxide (a colorless gas with a rotten-egg odor), are typically transformed into smaller, finer particulates, less than ten microns in diameter. Emitted mainly by coal- and oil-fired power plants, refineries, pulp and paper mills, and nonferrous smelters, they are a major contributor to acid rain, and are also filtered through the sinuses. Unfortunately, there is a price to be paid for protecting the lungs from this toxic substance. Sulfur oxide particles easily penetrate the mucosal lining. Studies have shown that they have an intensely irritating effect on the bronchial mucosa, resulting in damage to the cilia and initiation of bronchitis. If sulfur oxides can cause bronchitis in the lungs, would it be a far-fetched assumption that they can also cause sinusitis?

According to the EPA's 1988 National Air Quality and Emissions Trends Report, the metropolitan areas with the highest average particulate concentrations that year were, in descending order, Riverside–San Bernardino, California; St. Louis, Missouri; Tucson, Arizona; Los Angeles–Long Beach, California; and Las Vegas, Nevada. Those with the highest amounts of sulfur dioxide were Steubenville, Ohio; Weirton, West Virginia; Pittsburgh, Pennsylvania; New York City; Salt Lake City, Utah; and Evansville, Indiana.

Nitrogen oxides are the most obvious components of smog, providing color to the noxious cloud of air pollution. Their principal constituent is nitrogen dioxide, a yellowish-brown, highly reactive gas. Nitrogen oxides form when fuel is burned at high temperatures. The two major emission sources are internal combustion engines—motor vehicles and aircraft—and stationary fuel combustion sources such as electric utilities and industrial boilers. Like sulfur oxides, nitrogen oxides can irritate the lungs, causing ciliary paralysis, bronchitis, and pneumonia. They are also capable of impairing the body's immune defenses against bacterial and viral infection.

Los Angeles County is the only area in the country exceeding the federal nitrogen dioxide standard. The other cities that are highest in this pollutant are Riverside–San Bernardino, California; Anaheim, California; Denver, Colorado; Philadelphia, Pennsylvania; and Memphis, Tennessee.

Hydrocarbons are evaporated or incompletely burned organic compounds. The largest sources of hydrocarbons in the atmosphere include internal combustion engines; certain industrial processes, such as coke ovens in steel mills; and evaporation of liquids, such as gasoline in fuel transfers, and industrial and household solvents. Hydrocarbons are known to be highly irritating to the mucous membrane.

Ozone is the most dangerous component of smog. It is produced when sunlight acts upon nitrogen oxides and hydrocarbons. The many sources of both of these substances have already been mentioned. Ozone in the lower, breathable part of the atmosphere (within 1,000 feet of the earth's surface) is harmful to human and animal health, crops, and forests. In the upper atmosphere, ozone is beneficial, absorbing the harmful rays (ultraviolet-B) of sunlight. The continuing depletion of the upper ozone layer has become a serious health concern. Unfortunately, harmful ozone in the lower air does not move up to replenish the deteriorating ozone layer in the higher reaches of our atmosphere.

Ozone in the lower atmosphere is one of our greatest environmental challenges. Few, if any, urban areas are free of it. Four broad geographic regions are seriously affected: Southern California (by far the worst), the Northeast (especially the New York City area), the Texas Gulf Coast, and the Chicago–Milwaukee area. Cities with the worst ozone pollution are Los Angeles–Long Beach, Riverside–San Bernardino, and Anaheim–Santa Ana in California; Houston, Texas; and Bridgeport–Milford, Connecticut.

A growing body of scientific data indicates that ozone is a significant risk to human health, affecting not only those with impaired respiratory systems, such as asthmatics, but many with healthy lungs, both children and adults. Ozone can cause shortness of breath and coughing during exercise in healthy adults and more serious effects in the young, old, and infirm. Almost all of the research on ozone's effects has been done on lungs. There has not been any direct research on ozone and the sinuses. At the Air Pollution Health Effects Laboratory at the University of California, Irvine, however, its effects on the nasal cavities of rats have been studied. The findings lend substantial support to the connection between ozone and sinus disease. The researchers found significant damage to the mucous membrane surrounding the opening to the maxillary sinuses as a result of inhaling ozone. This could easily lead to the obstruction of the sinuses and subsequent infection. Robert Phalen, Ph.D., director of the laboratory, has also affirmed that "exposure to particulate pollution over a lifetime, can be associated with increased infection and more exposure to diseases."

Nowhere in the United States is the problem of air pollution more acute than in Los Angeles. A recent study on a group of that city's ten- and eleven-year-olds revealed that their lung capacity is already diminished by 17 percent compared to the normal range for that age. A pathologist at the University of Southern California, in performing autopsies on Los Angeles children killed accidentally, is finding a disturbing frequency of emphysematous changes previously seen only in adult lungs. But Los Angeles is not unique. Other areas of the country are well on their way to matching that city's severity of pollution and its damaging effects on the lungs and sinuses. There are also many agricultural communities that claim to be sinus "capitals" as a result of the pesticides and fertilizers that fill the air. I've heard from people in South Dakota, southern Minnesota, Iowa, North Carolina, and California's San Joaquin Valley, all reporting that "everyone has sinus problems."

Most physicians rate air pollution second only to cigarettes as a cause of the dramatic increase in the incidence of asthma, emphysema, chronic bronchitis (all have increased by 50 percent since 1981), and lung cancer. Americans are certainly not alone in suffering with this plague of pollution. According to the World Health Organization, residents of New Delhi, India; Seoul, Korea; and Mexico City breathe far worse air than that in Los Angeles. Dying forests across central Europe are a testament to the air pollution of that heavily industrialized continent. Huge demonstrations demanding a cleanup of air pollution have been reported in many Soviet cities.

There are solutions, of course, but most entail a change in lifestyle. In 1950, there were 50 million cars worldwide, 75 percent of them in the United States. This number doubled by 1960, redoubled by 1970, and doubled again by 1990—an eightfold increase to 400 million cars. American drivers now own only one-third of the world's total, but half of us have two cars in our garages. We have created a monster and it is killing us and the planet we live on. Automobiles, trucks, and buses are the chief sources of our air pollution. The availability and use of alternative fuels—ethanol, methanol, hydrogen, and natural gas—or the electric car would make a profound difference. Greater enforcement of engine emission tests, development of mass transit systems, participation in carpooling, and construction of bicycle paths, along with the conversion of power plants from coal to natural gas, the development of solar energy, and a reduction in wood burning—all would have an immediate impact on cleaning our air.

Many of us are already suffering the ill effects of breathing unhealthy air. A recent EPA study concludes that air pollution is responsible for approximately 60,000 deaths a year, making it one of the leading causes of death in the United States. In a landmark eleven-year study just completed by the UCLA School of Medicine, it was proven that irreversible lung deterioration can result from chronic exposure to polluted air. According to the American Lung Association, annual medical costs associated with human exposure to all outdoor air pollutants from all sources range from $40 billion to $50 billion. If each of us will do at least one thing to decrease air pollution, collectively we can cure this plague of unhealthy air.

AIR POLLUTION: INDOOR

Unfortunately, we cannot escape dirty air by remaining indoors. In 1988 the EPA reported that indoor air can be as much as 100 times more polluted than outdoor air, noting that Americans spend 90 percent of their time indoors. All of the indoor air pollutants listed in Table 1 have been proved harmful to the respiratory tract. Some of these pollutants originate in outdoor air.

Sick building syndrome is an unscientific term used to describe a pattern of disease symptoms linked to poor indoor air quality in workplaces, schools, homes, and other buildings. A sick building is one in which at least 20 percent of the occupants experience discomfort traceable to contaminated indoor air. Nationwide, as many as 80 million buildings might be of this type. Nearly a fifth of the work force in the United States has reported indoor air pollution ailments, ranging from headaches and fatigue to colds, influenza, and chronic respiratory illnesses (e.g., chronic sinusitis and chronic bronchitis). One million hospital visits a year are attributed to poor indoor air quality.

The EPA's own building in Washington, D.C., ironically, serves as an excellent example of sick building syndrome. More than a thousand of the 5,500 employees at EPA headquarters have complained of headaches, rashes, nausea, fatigue, blurred vision, chills, sneezing, fever, irritability, forgetfulness, hoarseness, dizziness, and burning sensations in their throats, ears, eyes, and chests. One employee commented, "I was afraid I was going to die in the place." Several of these symptoms can be attributed to sick sinuses and chronically inflamed respiratory tracts.

TABLE 1
INDOOR AIR POLLUTANTS

Combustion Products

Tobacco smoke

Coal- or wood-burning fireplaces and stoves

Fuel combustion gases from gas-fired appliances
such as ranges, clothes dryers, water heaters,
and fireplaces (they produce nitrogen dioxide,
carbon monoxide, nitrous oxides, sulfur oxides,
hydrocarbons, and formaldehyde)

Particulates

Dust

Pollen

Particles (frayed materials)

Asbestos

Chemicals and Chemical Solutions (chemicals that
affect indoor air quality are those associated
with architecture, the interior, artifacts, and
maintenance)

Fungicides and pesticides in carpet-cleaning
residues and sprays

Formaldehyde used in the manufacture of
insulation, plywood, fiberboard, furniture, and
wood paneling

Toxic solvents in oil-based paints, finishes,
coatings, and wall sealants

Aerosol sprays

Office equipment chemicals (photocopiers and
computers are common offenders, causing
chronic headaches and fatigue)

TABLE 1 *(continued)*

INDOOR AIR POLLUTANTS

Microorganisms (primarily from humidifiers, air
conditioners, and any other building components affected by excessive moisture)

Bacteria

Viruses

Molds (these are most prevalent in excessively
humid climates, such as Florida and the Gulf
Coast states, and are a primary cause of sinus
problems in those areas)

Dust mites

Radionuclides
Radon, a radioactive gas emitted from the earth
that enters homes primarily through basements,
crawl spaces, and water supply, especially from
wells (it can attach to the particulates of cigarette
smoke, dust particles, and natural aerosols)

Automotive Fumes
Sources include outdoor traffic, outdoor parking
lots, and outdoor loading and unloading spaces,
as well as indoor garages

A major explanation for the sick building syndrome, experts say, is the nationwide campaign, which emerged during
the energy crisis of the mid-1970s, to conserve energy by sealing and insulating buildings. The tight, energy efficient homes
and buildings that evolved have a relatively low energy demand, but a correspondingly low ventilation rate. The demise
of the operable-window building and the replacement of natural ventilation with mechanical ventilation have diminished

the flow of fresh air, trapping pollutants inside. Furthermore, the fresh air in most cities is anything but fresh. There has also been an increase in the use of energy efficient heating and air-conditioning systems, which has often led to increased circulation of polluted indoor air. Another factor in the deterioration of indoor air quality is the type of materials used to construct and furnish buildings. Building materials and furniture made of petrochemical-based products and materials that can emit harmful chemical vapors over long periods of time are used in place of nonpolluting natural materials and fibers.

The EPA has spent hundreds of thousands of dollars trying to solve the problem of its sick headquarters, but the symptoms continue. There is, however, a great deal that can be done to improve indoor air quality. Chapter 8 will offer some suggestions.

DRY AIR

An important function of the sinuses is to humidify the air we breathe; a person with weak sinuses may therefore have a problem in especially dry air. Moist air, that between 40 and 60 percent humidity, is very helpful for the proper functioning of the mucous membrane, especially the cilia. Dry air is usually found in conjunction with

- arid or semiarid climate;
- forced-air heating systems (they not only dry, but give the sinuses more to filter);
- air conditioning, especially in cars;
- oxygen therapy for various respiratory conditions;
- wind;
- mountains (the higher the elevation, the drier the air); and
- wood-burning stoves.

Dry air is hard on sinuses, but excessively moist air can also cause problems. Many microorganisms, such as bacteria, viruses, and molds, thrive when the humidity exceeds 60 percent.

COLD AIR

Although the moisture content of cold air is generally much higher than that of dry air, the shock of cold temperatures to the mucous membrane of an impaired sinus can cause significant irritation and ciliary injury, and often results in at least a runny nose. The least stressful air temperatures are between 65° and 85°F.

ALLERGIES

Those with asthma and nasal allergies, also called hay fever, are very susceptible to sinus infections. Their nasal and sinus mucosae are extremely sensitive and often hyperactive and potentially hypersecretory. When an allergic reaction takes place there is swelling of the mucosa and obstruction of the sinuses. Although the theory is untested, I strongly believe that chronic breathing of polluted air heightens the sensitivity of the nasal mucosa, hence creating an increasing number of new allergy sufferers and worsening the allergic condition of many others.

Many people claim that they are "allergic" to cigarette smoke, or dust, or some other irritant in the air. Most of the time they are not really describing an allergy, but rather an extreme irritation of the mucous membrane. This sensitivity causes a similar end result, nasal stuffiness and mucus drainage, but the process is a bit different. Actual nasal allergies are usually caused by airborne pollen from grass, trees, weeds, and flowers; molds; and dander from cats, dogs, horses, or other animals. In many areas of the United States, especially in parts of California and Florida where there is something pollinating year-round, allergies are the major contributors to sinus problems. Be aware, however, that if you are complaining of a year-round allergy problem, you might have chronic sinusitis.

In recent years an increasing number of physicians have become nutrition oriented, and are recognizing that food allergies might be a factor in chronic sinusitis. The foods most often implicated are wheat, cow's milk and all other dairy products, chocolate, corn, soy, white sugar, yeast (both brewer's and baker's), oranges, tomatoes, bell peppers, white potatoes, eggs, garlic, peanuts, black pepper, red meat, coffee, black tea, beer, wine, and champagne.

OCCUPATIONAL HAZARDS

A job performed in dirty, dry, and extremely hot or cold air should be considered a high risk to the sinuses. In my experience, those at highest risk include

- auto mechanics,
- construction workers (especially carpenters, who are America's highest-risk group for ethmoid sinus cancer),
- painters,
- beauticians,
- airport and airline personnel (mechanics, maintenance workers, baggage handlers, flight attendants, and even pilots),
- white-collar workers in offices where there are one or more smokers,
- policemen,
- firemen,

- parking garage attendants, and
- professional cyclists (the highest-risk group; they have more air to filter and are exposed to extremely cold, dry, and often dirty air).

When I worked as the team physician for the 7-Eleven cycling team during the 1986 Coors International Bicycle Classic, a total of five riders in the competition, including Eric Heiden of 7-Eleven, had to drop out because of sinus infections—this in spite of the fact that professional cyclists are the most physically fit human beings I have ever known.

DENTAL PROBLEMS

The roots of the teeth and the maxillary sinus are in close proximity; they are separated only by paper-thin bone or sinus mucosa. Because of this proximity, periapical abscesses or periodontitis of the upper teeth can extend into the sinus cavity and cause maxillary sinusitis. Minor trauma or injury, dental instrumentation, extraction, or displacement of a chronically inflamed tooth can lead to perforation of the sinus cavity. The incidence of dental-related sinusitis in children is unknown but probably significant, particularly in adolescents. In adults, possibly 10 percent of maxillary sinus infections are thought to be of dental origin.

IMMUNODEFICIENCY

The immune system is the human body's natural defense against infection, cancer, or inflammation; indeed, any form of illness. Sometimes, for reasons medical science has been unable to explain, the immune system does not function normally. Vital components of this system are infection-fighting

Save 40¢

ON ANY

Carefree

PANTY SHIELDS

(Not good on Trial Size)

Available in Original, Scented, Unscented and Longs

40¢

40¢

MANUFACTURER'S COUPON | NO EXPIRATION DATE

Carefree

PANTY SHIELDS

Carefree Longs®

Carefree

Save 40¢

ON ANY

Stayfree®

PRODUCT

(Not good on Trial Size)

40¢

Absorbs Your Worries
About Accidents And Odor

The ARM & HAMMER ® logo and the words ARM & HAMMER are trademarks of Church & Dwight Co., Inc.

40¢

MANUFACTURER'S COUPON | NO EXPIRATION DATE

Stayfree®

PANTY LINER 22 Pack

LIGHT DAYS AND EVERYDAY

WITH ODOR ABSORBING

Coupon 1 (Carefree)

Save 40¢ ON ANY

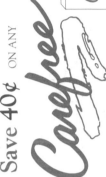

Carefree

PANTY SHIELDS
(Not good on Trial Size)

Available in Original, Scented, Unscented and Longs

Limit one coupon per purchase. Personal Products Company will reimburse you for the face value of this coupon plus 8¢ handling if submitted in compliance with Personal Products Coupon Redemption Policy CRP-1. Copies available upon request. Send coupons to: PERSONAL PRODUCTS COMPANY, Box #870082, El Paso, TX 88587-0082.

5 08004 10040 0
981802

Coupon 2 (Stayfree)

MANUFACTURER'S COUPON | NO EXPIRATION DATE

Save 40¢ on Super Long, Super, Regular, Deodorant, Thin, Mini, Panty Liner or Ultra Plus

(except Trial Size)

Stayfree®

Absorbs Your Worries
About Accidents And Odor

Limit one coupon per purchase. Personal Products Company will reimburse you for the face value of this coupon plus 8¢ handling if submitted in compliance with Personal Products Coupon Redemption Policy CRP-1. Copies available upon request. Send coupons to: PERSONAL PRODUCTS COMPANY, Box #870082, El Paso, TX 88587-0082.

5 08004 90040 6
981794

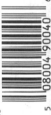
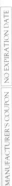

proteins called immunoglobulins. In immunodeficiency there is a decrease in the amount of one or two of these proteins. This condition can be diagnosed by a blood test. People who have a hereditary predisposition to it, who are on a course of chemotherapy, or who are taking cortisone long-term for a chronic condition are likely to have impaired immune systems. Most often, however, there is no known cause. I have observed for some time that people who have had long-term or repeated courses of antibiotic therapy appear to have very weak immune systems. These people are extremely prone to recurrent sinus infections.

MALFORMATIONS

Malformations include any physical problem that would result in the obstruction of the tiny sinus openings, the ostia. The most common malformations are a deviated septum (the wall that divides the two sides of the nose), enlarged adenoids (especially in young children), and polyps, cysts, or turbinate hypertrophy (swelling of the mucosal lining covering the internal nasal ridges).

EMOTIONAL STRESS

Emotional stress is probably the single most important determinant in whether someone develops a sinus infection. All of the other factors described in this chapter have the potential to adversely affect the sinuses, but what is it that triggers that potential? Why is it that a person with weak sinuses can be exposed to the same "risky" conditions many times but only occasionally develop a sinus infection? I am convinced that the answer is usually stress.

In the past few years, the new science of psychoneuroimmunology has legitimized the old notion that thoughts and emotions can both cause and combat disease. Recent research has provided a wealth of information on the profound impact our thoughts, beliefs, feelings, and attitudes have on our immune system and on our health. This knowledge is not new to holistic medicine. You will find its application to the treatment of sinus disease in Part II.

3 RECOGNIZING A SICK SINUS: ACUTE AND CHRONIC

Throughout this book I use the term *sinusitis* to refer to sinus problems in general. This word actually means "inflammation of a sinus" and encompasses two distinctly different medical diagnoses: acute sinusitis and chronic sinusitis.

ACUTE SINUSITIS

Acute sinusitis is another way of saying sinus infection. This is the problem that usually requires medical attention. I have already mentioned that the common cold is most often the cause of a sinus infection, so let's look at this a bit more closely.

A person who has had negligible or no sinus problems previously will notice that after seven to ten days a cold still won't quit, or that the cold symptoms have actually gotten much worse, or that the cold was almost gone for one or two weeks and now it's back again. Close questioning reveals that the "cold" never really went away.

In people whose sinuses have been weakened by previous infections, the common cold causes problems much sooner. These patients might notice the symptoms of a sinus infection within two or three days of the onset of the cold. The underlying condition of the sinuses will usually determine how soon the symptoms appear. Keep in mind that a common cold very often precedes the onset of acute sinusitis. Its appearance in the history of one's illness will help in the diagnosis of acute sinusitis. The most common symptoms follow. Note that the symptoms might differ for children under age twelve.

Head Congestion

Most people describe this symptom as fullness or a stuffy head. The nose might be stuffy as well. This symptom is most obvious in the morning upon arising from bed. It is often relieved, although not eliminated, by a hot shower. Voice, smell, and taste might be altered. These symptoms, however, are more subtle than the primary one of head congestion. There is a very definite awareness of a fullness in the head or a dull ache behind or above the eyes. *Dizziness* and *lightheadedness* are other words that might be used to describe this symptom.

Headache and Facial Pain

I have combined these two symptoms because it is often difficult to differentiate between them. With acute sinusitis, pain, and sometimes swelling, will occur in the region of the affected sinus (Figure 5). This usually results from air, pus, and mucus being trapped within the obstructed sinus. An infected maxillary sinus will cause pain, and sometimes swelling, in the cheek. Pain might occur under the eye and in the teeth of the upper jaw, particularly the molars. At times, the tooth pain can be so severe as to prompt a visit to the dentist. When air is prevented from entering a sinus by a swollen mucous membrane at its opening, a vacuum can be created, also resulting in severe pain in the affected sinus.

Infected ethmoid sinuses produce pain between and behind the eyes, and tenderness when pressure is applied to the sides of the nose. Infected frontals cause pain in the forehead

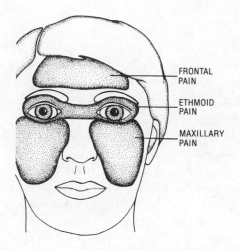

FIGURE 5   *Location of Sinus Pain in Acute Sinusitis*

and over the eyes. Infected sphenoids produce a generalized pain, deep in the head, which becomes aggravated whenever your head is jarred. Sphenoid pain is often perceived as a headache in the back of the head at the base of the skull.

Children might experience facial pain accompanied by swelling of the orbit of the eye that involves the upper eyelid. Gradual in onset, the swelling is most obvious in the early morning, shortly after rising. The swelling might decrease or even disappear during the day, only to reappear the following day. Children might also experience photophobia, which is an unwillingness to open the eyes in bright light.

Some of the most incapacitating headaches I have seen resulted from infected frontal sinuses. Sinus headaches tend to worsen when you bend your head forward or lie down, and tend to be worse in the morning, after you have been in bed for hours, and then ease somewhat later in the day.

Extreme Fatigue

There is scarcely a sinus patient I can think of who doesn't complain of some degree of fatigue. Most people, even if they are not ill, would admit to being tired for some part of the day. The word *extreme* in regard to fatigue means a definite change in normal energy level.

In addition to inquiring about the nasal and head symptoms that are usually mentioned by the patient, I always ask the questions, "Does your whole body feel sick in some way?" and "Do you feel especially tired?" The answer to these questions is frequently yes because acute sinusitis is usually a systemic illness, one that affects the entire body. These patients are sick all over. The medical term that best describes this phenomenon is *malaise*, meaning a feeling of general discomfort. It is often accompanied by significant irritability. People with sinus infections are usually sleeping more at night than they normally would, having some difficulty getting through a full day at work, and perhaps even taking unaccustomed naps. In people who exercise regularly, the drop in energy level is even more evident.

At times, fatigue is the chief complaint. The bad cold someone had was as long ago as two or three months, and they say, "I just haven't been myself since." These people do not come in complaining of the cold they still have; most of the time they think they are finished with it. If asked, however, they will admit to a stuffy head in the morning and occasional yellow mucus they have to spit out. These patients pose a tough diagnostic challenge to the physician, as some of them have been tired for so long they have no recollection of any previous illness. Others have been misdiagnosed with anything from depression to menopause. A few days of antibiotics, however, can do what months of estrogen were unable to do.

Yellow Mucus

The question that seems to make patients most uncomfortable is "What color is your mucus?" The usual response, accompanied by a grimace, is "Eww, I never look at it!" The classic presentation of acute sinusitis in children, infrequently seen in an adult, is yellow (actually a yellow-green) mucus coming from one nostril. If it's not (no pun intended), the diagnosis may be difficult. Most kids are not great nose-blowers, but sniffing actually makes matters worse, in that it tends to suck bacteria into the sinus. I usually try to have young patients blow their noses in the examination room. If you are checking your child at home, please remember to use white tissues; yellow won't help at all. Sinusitis is often missed in children. In fact, a recent article in a pediatric journal stated that almost 25 percent of all diagnosed upper respiratory tract infections (the common cold) in kids were actually cases of acute sinusitis.

In adults, yellow mucus from the nose will help make the diagnosis. However, in many cases the mucus is either clear or white, or there is none at all from the nose. It seems that in most adult cases of acute sinusitis the infected or yellow mucus drains down the back of the throat. People are most aware of this in the morning, when they get out of bed and spit into the sink some of the mucus their sinuses have produced during the night. This morning mucus is helpful in making the diagnosis, but it can also be present in the absence of acute sinusitis. Therefore, the most important question I ask an adult is, "Are you spitting out yellow mucus during the rest of the day, other than first thing in the morning?" Unfortunately, most people will respond with "I swallow it," or "It's not convenient to spit it out," or the old standby, "I never look at it!" If I still suspect a sinus infection, I will ask if they are even aware of mucus dripping down the back of the throat. If they're not aware of this occurring during the day, I then ask, "How about when you wake up in the morning?" Often I see patients who aren't aware of mucus drainage, but when I look at their throats, there is a thick yellow band of mucus running down from their sinuses.

I've spent a lot of time on the topic of mucus not because I enjoy discussing "gross" subjects, as my daughter Julie would say, but because it is extremely helpful in making the diagnosis. There are very few objective, or visible, signs of acute sinusitis, but this one is consistently present.

Refining the Diagnosis

Most ear, nose, and throat (ENT) specialists would find yellow mucus too indefinite a finding with which to make a diagnosis. Until 1986, they usually attempted to confirm the diagnosis with a sinus X-ray. However, this is unreliable. Some patients will have every symptom of a sinus infection although an X-ray shows a normal sinus.

In the past several years, new technology has made the definitive diagnosis of acute sinusitis much more feasible. The CT ("cat") scan, a computerized tomographic X-ray technique, can show areas of the sinuses never clearly visible with conventional X-rays. As a result, the diagnosis of sinus disease, and correspondingly, the statistics on its incidence, have risen dramatically. Unfortunately, the average sinus CT scan is costly.

To help reduce medical costs—as well as to assist primary care physicians, allergists, and ENT specialists in treating sinus infections—it would be a great advantage to have a generally accepted clinical diagnosis of acute sinusitis. This is what I offer here: a list of signs and symptoms that are so often present with sinus infections that they will preclude the need for X-rays and other expensive diagnostic procedures.

The picture presented by acute sinusitis can vary greatly; some people are very sick, others minimally uncomfortable. However, you can usually depend on these elements to make a definitive clinical diagnosis in an adult: a preceding cold, head congestion, headache, extreme fatigue, and postnasal yellow mucus. In a child the most common symptoms are nasal yellow mucus, fever, foul-smelling breath, and cough.

More Diagnostic Clues

The following symptoms are not quite as consistent as the foregoing, but are frequently present.

Fever A high temperature accompanying sinusitis is much more common in children than in adults. When fever is present in an adult, it is usually less than 101°F. It is not uncommon to see kids run high fevers (as high as 103° to 105°F) with acute sinusitis. Fever often appears early in the course of the infection—when other symptoms are not yet obvious—making the diagnosis difficult. Because fever accompanies so many different infections, it can't be considered an important diagnostic symptom. However, if I suspect sinusitis, fever, along with the other symptoms, can be a helpful sign in confirming the diagnosis.

Nasal Congestion and Rhinorrhea A stuffy and runny nose (rhinorrhea) is a primary symptom of the common cold that usually precede acute sinusitis. The two infections often overlap. The important thing to remember in adult sinusitis is that stuffiness is more common than a runny nose and is often present on only one side of the nose. In children with sinusitis, the yellow nasal discharge can be copious. With a cold, draining mucus is usually clear or white and thin or watery. With sinusitis it is usually thick and yellow.

Sore Throat   A sore throat is probably the most common complaint in any family doctor's office. The underlying problem is not always sinusitis, but a substantial number of sore throats do result from mouth breathing and from postnasal mucus drainage down the back of the throat. A sore throat from sinusitis is usually not consistent throughout the day; it is much worse in the morning upon awakening. In fact, the soreness, caused by constant postnasal mucus drainage, a stuffy nose, and mouth breathing can keep people from sleeping through the night. The dry air most of us breathe in our bedrooms can be irritating, too. Once I have established that a patient's sore throat is much worse first thing in the morning, I ask if the patient is aware of mucus draining down the back of the throat. (In children, this drainage often results in bad breath.) After that, I merely have to run through a checklist of the other sinus symptoms—mucus color, recent cold, fatigue, fever, and so on—to decide if this is sinusitis or something else. Most of these questions would be asked as part of a thorough investigation of any sore throat.

Laryngitis   Laryngitis, or hoarseness, is another common symptom of sinus infection. It results from the same factors that cause sore throat, primarily postnasal mucus draining down into the larynx, causing irritation, inflammation, and swelling of the vocal cords and the arytenoid cartilages in the larynx.

Cough   For most of the patients who come to a family doctor's office with a sinus infection, cough and sore throat are the symptoms that have resulted in the greatest discomfort and the most loss of sleep. Unfortunately, they are also the symptoms that have resulted in the highest number of misdiagnoses. A cough might be mistaken for bronchitis. Why? Because the cough of a sinusitis patient comes from yellow mucus draining down the back of the throat and continuing into the trachea or upper airway. Most physicians are aware that a productive cough that brings up a purulent or yellow mucus is often bronchitis. It isn't unusual to make that diagnosis in spite of hearing clear lungs with the stethoscope. It is easy to understand this common mistake, but it is just as easy to ask a few simple questions to rule out bronchitis and rule in acute sinusitis.

The cough from a sinus infection in adults isn't usually too bad during the day, when they are upright, but often worsens as soon as they lie down in bed at night. In children, the cough tends to be persistent throughout the day, just as it is in adults with bronchitis. Adults usually swallow the postnasal mucus drainage unconsciously, while up and about. This gets the mucus away from the trachea and into the stomach. (Swallowing the mucus can result in another not uncommon symptom that accompanies sinus infections: gastrointestinal upset; i.e., abdominal discomfort and loose bowels. There might be two or three loose movements a day—not quite diarrhea, but a definite change in bowel pattern. However, this isn't nearly as common as other symptoms I've mentioned, so I apologize for getting off the tract—respiratory, that is. Now, back to the cough.)

After asking about the timing of the cough, I usually want to know, "Does the cough feel like it's deep in your chest or does it feel more like a tickle in the back of your throat?" The latter, a dry cough, is much more typical of sinusitis; whereas the former, a wet, mucusy cough, is more indicative of bronchitis. In the past few years, I have noticed a definite increase in the number of patients who are infected simultaneously in the sinuses and lungs. This is called sinobronchitis. If the antibiotic treatments for sinusitis and bronchitis were the same, there would be no need to differentiate between the two. However, this is not the case, and I believe it is valuable to be as specific as possible in a treatment program.

I began this chapter by describing acute sinusitis as an infection usually requiring medical attention. A visit to the doctor has a twofold purpose: to diagnose the problem and to begin treating it. Ideally, there should also be a third objective: education and prevention. That is, teaching the patient how to care for his sinuses so that future office visits for the same problem will be unnecessary.

Again, the recognition of acute sinusitis is not a simple matter, even for physicians. Because the condition can manifest itself differently from one time to the next, this chapter and the next should be referred to frequently.

CHRONIC SINUSITIS

By now some of you might think the diagnosis of acute sinusitis is a piece of cake. Let me challenge you with the chronic variety. The National Center for Health Statistics says chronic sinusitis is the most common chronic disease in the United States. Although it affects nearly one of every seven Americans, many who have it couldn't tell you they do. Their situation is similar to that of the hundreds of thousands of people who are unaware they have high blood pressure and diabetes, two other common chronic conditions. Although they might not be able to attach a label to the problem, what these sinus sufferers are very familiar with are postnasal drip, congestion, headaches, fatigue, halitosis, and a weak sense of smell. These nuisances have been a part of their daily lives for years, and most have just accepted them.

Doctors have even more difficulty with this diagnosis than with acute sinusitis. They haven't paid much attention to chronic sinusitis because they don't consider it a disease that might shorten life expectancy.

Chronic sinusitis can be either a persistent, low-grade infection or a chronic inflammation of the mucosal lining of the nose and sinus cavities. I am seeing an increasing number of moderately to severely afflicted patients in the former category. They have taken repeated courses of antibiotics, often for more than a year. Some have had sinus surgery, with no significant positive effect. These individuals are extremely frustrated, often angry, and feel chronically ill. Their physicians share their exasperation. Medical science has done all it can do for them, and to no avail. I will call them group 1.

Other chronically infected people have accepted their condition as something they must live with. They might have been told by a physician, following an unsuccessful attempt at treatment, to give up hope, or they might be unaware that they have a medically treatable problem. Their infection usually persists in a low-grade state without becoming incapacitating. These people don't feel sick and have adjusted to their condition as their normal state of health. They are in what I will call group 2.

Group 2 is similar to what I will call group 3, patients with chronic sinus inflammation without infection. Inflammation involves pain, swelling, and increased secretions from the mucous membrane, but without the causative agents of bacteria, viruses, or fungi that are present in infection. People with an infection are usually sicker and weaker than those with inflammation only, and have a somewhat depressed immune system.

Groups 2 and 3 suffer less than group 1, but each group endures head congestion; nasal congestion; nasal and especially postnasal mucus drainage (often yellow in groups 1 and 2; white in group 3); headaches, irritability, and fatigue (especially in group 1); halitosis; and a diminished sense of smell and taste. Most chronic sufferers have an increased sensitivity to the factors mentioned in Chapter 2, such as smoke, pollution, pollen, dryness, cold, and fumes. The more they are exposed to any one of these irritants, the more pronounced the symptoms will be, and the more often these people are likely to develop acute sinus infections. For many of them, a routine common cold is rare. What starts out that way frequently develops into an acute sinusitis. Chronic infection decreases one's natural resistance, so almost any acute infection, whether it begins as influenza, strep throat, gastroenteritis (vomiting and diarrhea), or a number of other diseases, will often cause a sinus infection indirectly just by depressing an already weakened immune system.

Until recently, the diagnosis of chronic sinusitis has been difficult, relying almost entirely on the patient's description of his or her condition. An X-ray might reveal a thickened mucosa, but this is not necessarily diagnostic of sinusitis. In a small percentage of cases, a routine doctor's examination might show a deviated nasal septum or polyps that have blocked the sinus openings, the ostia. However, in the past few years, medical technology has developed a telescopic device called an endoscope. This flexible fiber-optic instrument can be inserted into the nose for a much clearer view of the areas of possible sinus blockage. The endoscope helps to confirm the diagnosis of chronic sinusitis and has been responsible for greatly improving the results of sinus surgery.

The vast majority of chronic sinus sufferers recognize that something isn't right, but they aren't sure why or what to do about it. For most, the condition began as a result of one or more episodes of acute sinusitis, repeated nasal allergies, or constant exposure to irritants such as cigarette smoke, pollution, or fumes. All can leave the sinuses in a permanently damaged state. Chronic sinusitis is not a life-threatening illness, but it affects its victims daily, poses a threat to the health of their lungs, and is an energy-draining condition that can have a profound impact on their ability to enjoy their lives.

4 TREATING ACUTE SINUSITIS

What does it mean to treat an ailment? This usually depends on what the condition is. In some instances, treatment implies a cure, with the expectation that the problem will not recur. These treatments are most often surgical. For example, appendicitis is treated with an appendectomy.

At other times, to treat means to relieve symptoms of a condition that has no known cure. These conditions range from cancer and AIDS to the common cold and sore throat. Relief of symptoms constitutes the bulk of a physician's work; almost 75 percent of all ailments fall into this treatment realm.

The treatment of acute sinusitis is in yet another category. Acute sinusitis is a bacterial infection in one or more of the sinus cavities. The goal of treatment is to kill the bacteria, open the blocked sinus duct, and restore the mucus-and-cilia cleansing system, while relieving symptoms. Acute sinusitis does have a cure, but the chances of its recurring at some point, either months or years later, are very high.

Acute sinusitis is not a simple infection to treat. Doctors seldom identify the bacteria that cause the infection, so they select an antibiotic to combat the bacteria most likely to have caused the infection. The antibiotic is taken by mouth and absorbed into the bloodstream. Because of the relatively poor blood supply in the sinuses, it usually takes several days before the effect of the drug is felt, especially in adults. Strong antibiotics in relatively high dosages taken for long periods of time are often required.

The next objective is to open the blocked sinus duct and the ostium so that the infected mucus can drain from the sinus. A decongestant opens the duct by shrinking the swollen mucous membrane. However, most decongestants have a drying effect, especially if used in combination with an antihistamine, probably because most commercial decongestants also contain an antihistamine. This drying will thicken the mucus and prevent it from draining.

Acute sinusitis is an infection without an accepted standard treatment program. Antibiotics have been, and continue to be, the primary component of the traditional medical treatment. However, if there was one drug that always worked for everyone, this would be a very brief discussion, and I would not have to devote an entire chapter to the subject. The reality is that the efficacy of treatment varies with each patient and with the physician who is administering the treatment. During the past decade, physicians have had to employ greater creativity, using a vastly expanded arsenal of antibiotics, decongestants, expectorants, nasal sprays, and antitussives to succeed in treating sinus infections.

ANTIBIOTICS

The bacteria most often responsible for causing sinus infections in both adults and children are *Streptococcus pneumoniae* and *Hemophilus influenzae*. Doctors have recently found a marked increase in the incidence of *Staphylococcus aureus*, especially in children, perhaps because of improved diagnostic techniques.

Unfortunately, the antibiotics that effectively treat all the bacteria that cause sinusitis are quite expensive. As sinus infections become more difficult to treat, especially those caused by *Staphylococcus aureus,* researchers come to the rescue with ever more powerful antibiotics.

For the past decade the drug of choice has been ampicillin or its more powerful variation, amoxicillin. The usual dosage of amoxicillin is either 250 or 500 mg (125 or 250 mg in children) three times a day. Both are taken for ten days. This is a routine first step, but it is a hefty dose of antibiotic! Adult patients are instructed that they will notice definite improvement, with the yellow mucus beginning to clear, in about four to five days. In children the response is usually faster, with fever, nasal drainage, and cough markedly reduced after about forty-eight hours. Patients are told to take the medicine for the entire ten days. If this instruction is not followed, the infection often remains. Many physicians routinely prescribe amoxicillin for fourteen days, instead of ten, to reduce the number of treatment failures. For the majority of patients with acute sinusitis, a ten-day course of amoxicillin is all they will need.

In spite of their compliance with instructions, 5 to 10 percent of patients will call or return to the office shortly after the tenth day, still complaining of most of their symptoms. Some will report that they felt much better while on the antibiotic, but that as soon as they stopped taking it the symptoms recurred. Others will say they experienced no improvement whatsoever, usually in a tone of voice that conveys the very clear message, "You'd better get rid of this infection real fast, or else." These are not my most amiable patients. Nor should they be. They have usually had the sinusitis for at least three weeks and have now made their second visit to the doctor.

With the second attempt at treatment, I almost always will choose a different antibiotic. The second-choice antibiotics have a bit broader spectrum of efficacy than amoxicillin; all are more expensive. Table 2 lists both amoxicillin and the second-step drugs that are commonly used for the treatment of acute sinusitis.

Most physicians have their own favorite second-step an-

TABLE 2
ANTIBIOTICS FOR ACUTE SINUSITIS

Brand Name & Quantity	Generic Equivalent	Strength/Average Dose	Adults (12+yr.) or Children	Average Price
	Amoxicillin Capsules #30	1) 250 mg 1 3X/day 2) 500 mg for 10 days	1) children 2) adults	1) $7 2) $9
	Amoxicillin Suspension 150 cc	250 mg/5 cc (1 tsp) 3X/dX10d	children	$7
Ceclor Capsules #30		250 mg 1 3X/dX10d		$48
Ceclor Suspension 150 cc		250 mg/5 cc 3X/dX10d	children	$41
Bactrim DS #20 or Septra DS	Trimethoprim- Sulfamethoxazole	1 2X/dX10d	adults	$22 $10 (generic)
Bactrim Suspension 200 cc	Trimethoprim- Sulfamethoxazole	10 cc (2 tsp) 2X/dX10d	children	$17 $9 (generic)
Vibramycin or Vibra-Tabs #20	Doxycycline	100 mg 1 2X/dX10d	adults	$56 $12 (generic)
Pediazole Suspension 200 cc	Erythromycin- Sulfisoxazole	5 cc 4X/dX10d	children	$26 $17 (generic)
Ceftin Tablets #20		250 mg 1 2X/dX10d	adults	$50
Cipro Tablets #20		500 mg 1 2X/dX10d	adults	$50
Suprax Tablets #10		400 mg 1X/dX10d	adults	$48
Suprax Suspension 100 cc		100 mg/5cc 1X/dX10d	children	$44

tibiotic, one with which they have seen the most therapeutic success and the fewest unpleasant side effects. Ceftin has replaced Ceclor as the popular choice. Both cost about $50 for a ten-day supply, but Ceftin seems to be more effective. It is taken twice a day, in a strength equivalent to Ceclor taken three times per day, and is easily absorbed with food.

A small but growing percentage of patients are still not cured following a ten-day course of a second-step antibiotic, or their infection returns again shortly after they finish. It sometimes helps to take a two- or even three-week course of the antibiotic and gradually taper it off over the last five to seven days. This seems to allow the body's immune system a better chance to take over for the antibiotic. Whatever the reason, this strategy does appear to be more effective than abruptly stopping the drug a patient has been taking for two to three weeks.

Patients who do not respond to antibiotics are good candidates for further diagnostic evaluation with an X-ray, CT scan, or rhinolaryngoscopy to see if there is a physical obstruction of the sinus. During the past year, however, I have seen several new patients without obstructions who have a history of nearly consecutive courses of different antibiotics over almost two years' time. It is true that these are extreme cases, but it appears that many physicians are being confronted with such problems. Since the first edition of *Sinus Survival* was published in November of 1988, three new "big gun" antibiotics are commonly being used as a last resort with stubborn sinus infections: Ceftin, Cipro, and Suprax. The latter, however, is ineffective against *Staphylococcus*. Their efficacy has been impressive, but how long can we continue to rely on the development of ever more powerful drugs?

DECONGESTANTS AND EXPECTORANTS

The decongestants are specifically used to open the ostia and sinus ducts while relieving the symptoms of head and nasal congestion, headache, facial pain, and, to some extent, sore throat and cough. Expectorants, which are mucus thinners, can help to relieve the same symptoms.

The challenge of using a decongestant is to find one whose benefits outweigh its side effects. Decongestants are readily available in many familiar over-the-counter (OTC) products, such as Dristan, Contac, Allerest, Drixoral, Actifed, Dimetapp, Triaminicin, and a host of other cold remedies. Every one of these contains an antihistamine in combination with the decongestant. This is also true of Sinutab and many other sinus remedies. Given the drying effect of antihistamines and the subsequent thickening of the mucus, I am convinced they do more harm than good. They are fine if all you are trying to treat is a cold, but I believe that in many instances they have actually helped a cold progress into a sinus infection.

If you have a history of sinus problems, I would advise you to avoid antihistamines. If you are not sure about the ingredients of an OTC product, ask a pharmacist.

The most common ingredients in both prescription and OTC decongestants are pseudoephedrine, phenylpropanolamine, and phenylephrine. Each works in much the same way to shrink swollen mucous membranes and reduce nasal and sinus congestion. Many products contain these decongestants in combination. Some, available only by prescription, include two of these ingredients; others only one, along with a pain reliever or an expectorant or cough suppressant.

There is a myriad of choices at the pharmacy. The following is a guide to lead you through the confusing maze of cold and sinus preparations. Before you begin the process, it would be helpful to ask yourself what it is you are treating. What are the symptoms that most trouble you? Are you stuffed up? Or is it the headache, the cough, the sore throat, or the thick mucus that you would most like to eliminate? Since you probably have more than one symptom, you will be looking for a decongestant in combination with something else. However, choose anything but an antihistamine. I recommend the preparations in tables 3 through 7. If all you need is a plain decongestant, then Sudafed tablets are an excellent choice. If you have a lot of thick mucus draining, don't want a decongestant, and would like a simple expectorant, Fenesin, Humibud, and Organidin are all good prescription drugs.

Tables 3, 4, and 7 all list OTC products. Please follow the dosage instructions on the bottle or package. The drugs in Table 5, which your doctor might prescribe, contain the same decongestants and expectorants as those found in the OTC products. The primary difference is that these drugs contain higher doses and are long-acting, continuing to work for up to twelve hours. The exceptions are Entex and Dura-Gest capsules, the latter of which is both a brand-name drug and used by most pharmacists as the generic form of Entex. These

TABLE 3
Decongestants with Analgesics (OTC)

Allerest No Drowsiness Tablets
Coldrine Tablets
Congesprin Cold Tablets for Children
Dristan Maximum Strength Caplets
Dristan Sinus Tablets
Fiogesic Tablets
Naldegesic Tablets
Ornex Caplets
St. Joseph Cold Tablets for Children
Sinarest No Drowsiness Tablets
Sine-Aid Maximum Strength Caplets
Sine-Aid Sinus Headache Tablets
Sine-Off Maximum Strength No Drowsiness
Formula Caplets
Sinus Excedrin Tablets and Caplets
Sinutab Maximum Strength Without Drowsiness
Caplets
Specification-T Sore Throat/Decongestant
Lozenges
Sudafed Maximum Strength Sinus Tablets and
Caplets
Super Anahist Tablets
Tylenol Maximum Strength Sinus Tablets and
Caplets

TABLE 4
DECONGESTANTS WITH EXPECTORANTS (OTC)

Robitussin-PE Syrup
Triaminic Expectorant

TABLE 5
DECONGESTANTS WITH EXPECTORANTS (Rx)

Dura-Gest Capsules
Dura-Vent Tablets
Entex Capsules
Entex LA Tablets
Entex Liquid
Guaifed Capsules
Guaifed-PD Capsules
Guaitab Tablets
Nolex LA Tablets
Respaire-60 SR Capsules
Respaire-120 SR Capsules
Respinol-LA Tablets
T-Moist Tablets
Tuss-LA Tablets
Zephrex LA Tablets

short-acting products can be taken every four to six hours and
contain two decongestants, phenylephrine and phenylpropanolamine, in combination with the expectorant guaifenesin. I
find them more effective in the treatment of acute sinusitis
than the long-acting preparations. Avoid them if you have high
blood pressure. They can cause insomnia in adults, but some
young children experience the opposite side effect and be-

come drowsy. Omitting the bedtime dose usually eliminates the insomnia.

I usually don't encourage patients to take the decongestant on the same rigid schedule as the antibiotic, or for the entire ten-day course. I tell them to take it regularly for the first four to five days, then gradually taper off. If they still experience head and sinus congestion, they should continue the ten-day course. Patients with active sinus infections should avoid air travel because of the pressure changes and poor air quality found on airplanes. If they can't, I recommend taking a decongestant approximately two hours prior to the scheduled landing.

DECONGESTANT SPRAYS

An OTC alternative for those with extreme head and nasal congestion or sinus pain is nasal decongestant spray. There are several twelve-hour varieties from which to choose, including Afrin, Dristan, Sinex, Neo-Synephrine, and Vicks. These should be used with great caution and only for two or three days at most. They can easily become addictive! They produce what is called a rebound effect, which means that as their decongestant effect wears off and the head and nasal congestion return, the feeling of stuffiness is worse than it was before using the spray. This elicits a strong desire to spray again, and a vicious cycle begins. Be careful!

If you have been using a spray regularly and are unable to stop, you probably need some help. Consult with your physician and tell him honestly what has been happening. I have had a high success rate helping patients to break this habit with the following regimen:

- Throw away the nasal spray.
- Take a tapered dose of cortisone over a one-week

period, either Medrol (the generic name is methyl-prednisolone) in the 4-mg dosepak or 5 mg of predni-sone. These are prescription drugs that relieve inflammation.

- Take forty capsules of Entex or Dura-Gest in a tapered schedule: one capsule three times a day over seven days; then one capsule two times a day over seven days; followed by one capsule daily before bed over seven days.
- Use moisture—including saline nasal spray, a humi-difier, and steaming in the bathroom (refer to this chapter's Moisture and Irrigation section)—as a decongestant measure.

Remember that it is extremely difficult to keep your si-nuses healthy with continued use of a decongestant nasal spray.

ANTITUSSIVES (COUGH SUPPRESSANTS)

If a patient's chief complaint is a cough that interrupts sleep, I will withhold the bedtime dose of decongestant and substi-tute a strong prescription cough suppressant containing either codeine or hydrocodone in combination with a decongestant, an expectorant, or both. Such antitussives can cause drowsi-ness, which is why I rarely recommend them for daytime use. Besides, these people are already tired from having a sinus in-fection. They don't need any additional sedation. The most commonly prescribed antitussives for sinus patients are listed in Table 6. If a cough suppressant is indicated for use during the day, especially in children, there are several similar OTC combination drugs from which to choose. They can be taken by both adults and children. These are listed in Table 7.

TABLE 6
ANTITUSSIVES WITH DECONGESTANTS OR EXPECTORANTS (Rx)

Detussin Expectorant

Donatussin DC Syrup

Hycomine Pediatric Syrup

Hycomine Syrup

Naldecon CX Liquid

Novahistine Expectorant

Nucofed Expectorant

Robitussin A-C

Robitussin-DAC

Triaminic Expectorant with Codeine

Tussend-DAC

Tussend Expectorant

Tussi Organidin

Tussi Organidin DM

ANALGESICS (PAIN RELIEVERS)

To relieve the frequent symptoms of headache, facial pain, and sore throat, I recommend the OTC pain relievers Advil and Nuprin. Both contain ibuprofen, which not only relieves pain but reduces inflammation. (To some extent, ibuprofen also can lower a fever.) Both pain relievers are dispensed in 200-mg tablets, and they are safe for *adults* in dosages of three or even four at a time if the pain is especially severe. This high dosage, however, should be taken with food, especially if there is a history of stomach ulcers.

Aspirin has the same effects as ibuprofen, but doesn't seem to be as strong. Tylenol and other acetaminophen-containing products are simply analgesics, with no effect on

TABLE 7
ANTITUSSIVES WITH DECONGESTANTS AND EXPECTORANTS (OTC)

Ambenyl D Decongestant Formula
Bayer Children's Cough Syrup
Benylin Expectorant Liquid
Cheracol D Cough Liquid
Comtrex Cough Formula
Contac Cough Formula Liquid
Contac Jr. Liquid
Dorcol Children's Cough Syrup
Formula 44D Decongestant Cough Mixture
Formula 44M Liquid
Naldecon DX Pediatric Drops
Naldecon DX Children's Syrup
Naldecon DX Adult Liquid
Naldecon EX Pediatric Drops
Naldecon Senior DX Liquid
Novahistine DXM Syrup
Robitussin-CF
Robitussin DM Cough Calmers Lozenges
Robitussin DM Syrup
Ru-Tuss Expectorant
Sudafed Cough Syrup
Vicks Children's Cough Syrup

the inflamed sinuses. However, if lowering a fever is the primary objective, both aspirin and Tylenol would be better choices. Any acetaminophen-containing product is the drug of choice for children with acute sinusitis.

MOISTURE AND IRRIGATION

Moisture helps empty the sinus of its thick, infected mucus, and in doing so helps restore normal cilial function and relieves nasal and head congestion, headache, sinus pain, and sore throat. Warm, moist air is best, and the easiest place to get it is in the bathroom. Simply close any doors and windows and turn the shower on hot to create steam. You then have the choice of either getting in the shower, after adjusting the temperature, of course, or just sitting and relaxing in the steam until you run out of hot water. Make a conscious effort to breathe through your nose. Hot towels applied over the face can also be helpful.

As most of us do not have an endless supply of hot water, making a steam room of the bathroom can be done only two or three times a day. What about the rest of the time? If you are staying home from work, your best source of moist air is a humidifier placed by your bed, with the bedroom door and windows closed. Most humidifiers are quiet and very effective in producing a moist environment in an enclosed space. They are available in pharmacies, department stores, and hardware stores under a variety of brand names. The ideal humidifier has probably not yet been designed. The cool-mist ultrasonics put out a fine mineral dust unless distilled water is used to fill them, and the new warm ultrasonics have a tendency to break down. Steam humidifiers or vaporizers can become quite hot, which could be a concern if you have small children. The ultrasonic humidifiers with a demineralizing component seem to have eliminated most problems. The Bionaire CM-3 or CM-4 appears to be a good choice. Most room humidifiers cost between $40 and $100. Whatever your choice, be sure the reservoir tank opening is large enough to allow for cleaning. Wipe it daily with vinegar water; otherwise it becomes a breeding ground for molds. During treatment for a sinus infection, the humidifier should be used every night while you sleep. The moisture is very helpful in relieving the infection's cough and sore throat during the night.

Assuming your environment is relatively dry, as indoor air tends to be during the winter months in most parts of the United States, you can provide moisture with a saltwater, also called saline, nasal spray. There are several commercial products available in pharmacies. You can make your own saline spray by mixing a ½ teaspoon of salt in an 8-ounce cup of lukewarm water and dispensing it from a spray bottle. Spray into each nostril while closing off the other nostril and simultaneously inhaling. This is nonaddictive and can be done as often as you like throughout the day. It has no negative side effects, except for the curious looks you will get from those wanting to know what in the world you are doing.

An even more effective way of moisturizing is saline irrigation. This procedure can result in dramatic relief from pain, in that it reduces swelling in the nasal passages, causing a reduction of pressure in the sinus. Saltwater sprays also irrigate; i.e., wash out some mucus, bacteria, and dust particles, while reducing swelling. However, they don't do it as well as the following irrigation methods, which should be done three to four times a day.

Mix the saline solution for irrigation fresh each day in one cup of lukewarm tap water. Add ¼ to ½ teaspoon of table salt and a tiny pinch of baking soda, thus making the solution close to normal body fluid salinity and pH. Irrigating with plain water is usually somewhat uncomfortable. Use the full cup of saline solution for each irrigation (one-half cup for each nostril), irrigating over the sink, with the head in an upright position, using one of the following methods, but in an upright position. Always blow your nose *very* gently after irrigating.

Method 1: Completely fill a large, all-rubber, ear syringe (available at most pharmacies) with saline solution. Lean over the sink, pinch one nostril closed, and insert the syringe tip just inside the open nostril, pinching the nostril around the tip. *Gently* squeeze and release the bulb several times to swish the solution around the inside of your nose. The solution will run out both nostrils and might also run out of your mouth. Repeat this for each nostril until one cup of saline solution is used, or until the solution is clear.

Method 2: Pour saline solution into the palm of your hand and sniff the solution up your nose, one nostril at a time.

Method 3: Use an angled nasal irrigator attachment (the Grossan nasal irrigator is available at some pharmacies) on a Water Pik appliance. Set the Water Pik at the lowest possible pressure and insert the irrigator tip just inside one nostril, pinching your nostril to form a seal. Irrigate with your mouth open, allowing the fluid to drain out either your mouth or nose. Repeat the procedure in the other nostril.

Method 4: For very small children, irrigate with ten to twenty drops of saline solution per nostril from an eyedropper.

If you are using a decongestant nasal spray, use it only *after* the saltwater nasal irrigations.

These methods obviously require more effort than the saline nasal sprays, but many patients comment on how much more helpful it is.

Another solution that has been effective in irrigation is called Alkalol. It is a mucus solvent and cleaner, and can be used with the saline solution in a 1:1 ratio (½ saline, ½ Alkalol) with all of the methods previously mentioned. You will probably have to ask your pharmacist to order it for you, as it is not usually available, but Alkalol is very inexpensive.

HYDRATION AND BED REST

In regard to a cold, you have often heard the advice to drink a lot of liquids and stay in bed. For acute sinusitis, this advice is good. I recommend at least eight to ten 8-ounce glasses of water daily. Avoid ice-cold drinks and anything containing caffeine, sugar, or alcohol.

As for resting, try to listen to your body and not push yourself. As a general rule, if you are waking up to an alarm clock you are not getting enough sleep. Allow your body to tell you how much sleep you need and adjust your bedtime accordingly. Rest as much as possible during the first five to seven days of treatment.

MISCELLANEOUS

Many physicians have their own special sinus remedies. Several that are frequently mentioned, but with which I have no personal experience, are a combination of topical caffeine and Ocean saline nasal spray; Argyrol, a silver solution used as an anti-infective drop in the nose; and Ichthyol at 20 percent in glycerin, applied as a nasal packing to open the ostia and sinus ducts and draw infected mucus out of the sinuses.

In many cases, acute sinusitis coexists as a silent partner with a more easily identifiable ailment. The most common instances are discussed in the next chapter. In these circumstances, sinus infections should be treated with the same methods that have been described in this chapter. For additional help in treating acute sinusitis in regard to diet, vitamins, herbs, and nutritional supplements, refer to Chapter 10.

5 ACUTE SINUSITIS WITH OTHER MEDICAL CONDITIONS

It is not uncommon to find acute sinusitis together with other conditions that also affect the respiratory tract. When this occurs, it is almost always the concomitant problem, not the sinus infection, that is most apparent to both physician and patient. Two of these conditions—the common cold and nasal allergies—precede the onset of acute sinusitis, whereas the others usually occur subsequent to the sinus infection.

THE COMMON COLD

This is the most frequent illness that accompanies sinusitis. If you suspect that you have a sinus infection, or if you are at high risk for getting one, avoid taking antihistamines for your cold. Every cold can be treated with the same methods I have recommended for acute sinusitis, with the exception of the antibiotic. If a sinus infection is present along with a cold, it should become obvious in seven to ten days.

ACUTE OTITIS MEDIA (MIDDLE EAR INFECTION)

This is commonly seen in children, and very often in conjunction with acute sinusitis. The bacteria that cause this infection are the same as those responsible for sinus infections. The position and anatomy of the eustachian tube, which drains the middle ear space, helps create the simultaneous infections. I once heard an ENT physician say that anytime he sees an adult with otitis media, that person *always* has an underlying acute sinusitis.

When otitis media is present, sinusitis might be ignored or even remain unrecognized. These patients are extremely uncomfortable, and their ear pain becomes the focus of attention for both doctor and patient. Young children will usually have a fever above 101°F. The treatment of otitis media can be exactly the same as that of acute sinusitis; therefore, if the diagnosis of sinusitis is missed, the sinus infection usually will get better anyway. In adults with otitis media, however, I would recommend more regular use of a decongestant than I would for children, and for a longer period of time (three times a day for at least ten days) than I would with sinusitis. This is because adults with middle ear infections routinely complain of "stuffiness" in their ears long after the pain has gone, even after two or three weeks.

Many young children have repeated episodes of acute otitis media, as often as four or five times a year. Family physicians and pediatricians are very familiar with this type of patient. In most of them, a cold quickly becomes a sinus infection, which then causes the ear infection. The average number of colds contracted per year in young kids is six, which often occasions several visits to the doctor, or even to emergency rooms, as ear infections often begin at night. Many of these pediatric patients require surgery to place tubes through the eardrums to facilitate drainage.

ALLERGIC RHINITIS (NASAL ALLERGY)

When allergies accompany sinusitis, or the patient suffering from allergy symptoms has a history of recurrent sinus infections, the condition becomes one of medicine's more challenging problems. Because allergy results in swelling and inflammation of the nasal mucous membrane and consequent blockage of the sinus ducts, it is important to treat these symptoms before conditions become opportune for a sinus infection. A persistent flare-up of a runny nose and cough, or difficulty controlling nasal congestion and postnasal drainage with the usual allergy therapy, might signal that a sinus infection has already begun.

Many people with seasonal allergic rhinitis, or hay fever, may get relief from OTC medications such as Dristan, Contac, Allerest, Drixoral, Actifed, Dimetapp, Triaminicin, Sudafed Plus, and many others. They are helpful primarily because they contain both antihistamines and decongestants. Chlortrimeton is also popular but contains no decongestant.

Classic antihistamines are wonderful drugs for the treatment of allergies, although they may cause drowsiness and thickening of mucus secretions. Seldane and Hismanal, two of the new-generation antihistamines, are exceptions. They are non-sedating, and do not cause thickening of the mucus. For this reason, I recommend them to allergy sufferers who are also prone to sinus infections. If you have allergies in conjunction with weak sinuses or a current sinus infection, avoid the OTC antihistamines.

Another option for treating nasal allergies in a sinus sufferer is to use the prescription sprays Nasalcrom, Beconase, Vancenase, Nasalide, and the newly released Nasacort. Nasalcrom is a topical mast cell stabilizer, which simply means that it prevents the allergic reaction from taking place and therefore prevents the swelling of the nasal mucous membrane. Beconase and Vancenase are topical cortisone nasal sprays with both antiallergic and anti-inflammatory effects. They are available both as liquid sprays and as freon-based, metered-dose inhalers. These nasal sprays work even better if used after nasal irrigation. Irrigation removes the mucus secretions so that the prescription spray does not sit on the mucus but hits the lining of the nose directly. The irrigation will also remove allergens such as pollen and particulates.

A seasonal allergy sufferer who also has a history of sinus infection should use the spray on a maintenance schedule throughout the season. The majority of people with hay fever are reacting either to tree pollen (March–May), grasses (May–July), or weeds (August–October). These seasons will vary according to your locale. Use of the spray not only provides effective relief for their symptoms, but may also prevent both the acute sinusitis and the drowsiness that OTC antihistamines can cause. Treatment with prescription nasal sprays is not, however, without side effects. Long-term use of cortisone sprays can cause chronic irritation, inflammation, and increased mucus secretion. This is less of a problem with the aqueous-based than the freon-based sprays.

In the humid southern states, molds can be a significant problem all year long. In situations when allergens are present year-round, I recommend using the sprays only during the most severe periods of allergic reaction. I would also suggest seeing an allergist who, with an evaluation that may include skin testing, might recommend allergy desensitization shots. For many allergy sufferers these can be quite helpful in producing an immunologic resistance so the patient can tolerate exposure to the allergens and minimize the need for any medicine. Chapters 8 and 10 contain additional information that should help you cope with continuous allergies.

If someone has an acute sinusitis along with allergic rhinitis, the patient should use the regular sinusitis treatment regimen in addition to Nasalcrom, the cortisone sprays, Seldane, or Hismanal. Some of these patients are so uncomfortable that I prescribe a short course of cortisone tablets.

BRONCHITIS

Sinobronchitis is acute sinusitis coexisting with acute bronchitis. Although it is being seen more often, sinobronchitis is still not a simple diagnosis to make. The primary complaint is usually a persistent (day and night), deep, wet, and yellow-mucusy cough, and is even more commonly found in patients who smoke. The usual symptoms of sinusitis are also present. Needless to say, these people feel worse than the typical acute sinusitis patient.

Worse yet are those whose bronchitis has turned into pneumonia, which is simply a more severe lung infection than bronchitis. These patients are quite sick, with a bad cough and often fever and chills.

Both lung infections usually can be diagnosed by listening to the lungs with a stethoscope; pneumonia can be confirmed with a chest X-ray. When a sinus infection is also present, it most likely preceded the lung condition. In fact, the postnasal drainage of infected mucus into the lungs may have caused the lung infection.

Following diagnosis is selection of an antibiotic that will cure both infections. If the sinusitis remains, it will be difficult to get rid of the infection in the lungs. It is for this reason that I will not choose to start treatment with erythromycin. Although erythromycin might be the best choice for the lungs, I have seen many instances in which it was ineffective in treating the sinuses. Several of the broad-spectrum antibiotics listed in Table 2 would be better choices. The rest of the treatment program for acute bronchitis is the same as that for sinusitis, with an emphasis on breathing warm moist air. People with chronic bronchitis can benefit from most of the therapeutic measures for chronic sinusitis described in Part II, along with postural drainage techniques.

ASTHMA

Another disease of the lungs affected by sinusitis is asthma. The National Jewish Center for Immunology and Respiratory Medicine in Denver, a research center for asthma and other respiratory diseases, noted in a 1989 study that more than two-thirds of patients with mild to severe asthma showed abnormalities on sinus X-rays. It was also reported that in asthmatic children with moderate to severe sinus abnormalities, treatment of their sinuses may improve their asthma. The study referred to a 1925 report that postulated four mechanisms explaining how sinus disease could cause asthma, conclusions not substantially different from those made in the 1987 study. Two of these mechanisms are postnasal drip of mucus into the lower airways, which either directly alters airway reactivity or causes airway inflammation, and nasal obstruction, which causes mouth breathing, aggravating the asthma through loss of heat and moisture in the lower airways, particularly if the air breathed is cold or dry.

The National Jewish Center primarily treats asthmatics whose condition is poorly controlled or who depend on cortisone to control the asthma. The center's study linking sinus disease to asthma described many patients who improved dramatically and were able to decrease their steroid requirements following treatment of their sinusitis. This has been demonstrated by other studies and is now a well-accepted principle in the treatment of asthma. If this holds true for the most severely afflicted asthmatics, it should also apply to anyone with mild to moderate asthma who experiences a flare-up or an exacerbation of the condition. If an obvious cause for the asthmatic episode is not present—such as the common cold, allergy, exercise, or emotional stress—and the wheezing can't be controlled with the usual medication, consider the possibility of a sinus infection.

The same message holds true for the other conditions described in this chapter: sinusitis is far more prevalent than most people imagine. A sinus infection might be subtle in its presentation, but when it accompanies another condition, it can have a profound impact on the course of the illness.

Most of those who suffer from a sinus infection will find the treatment program described in Chapter 4 effective both in relieving discomfort and in eliminating the infection. However, for the growing number of people who have had repeated episodes of acute sinusitis and are now chronic sinus sufferers, for those who are seeking an alternative to the traditional medical approach, and for anyone interested in preventive medicine and in understanding how lifestyle contributes to sinus disease, Part II will be your next step to better health.

PART II

THE HOLISTIC APPROACH TO SINUSITIS

6 A REVIEW OF THE TRADITIONAL APPROACH

In Part II we will be looking at the holistic approach that has proven remarkably successful in the treatment of chronic sinusitis. Before beginning that discussion, I would like to review the options that traditional medicine offers, some of which you have undoubtedly tried. The conventional treatment for chronic sinusitis consists primarily of antibiotics and surgery, medicine's biggest guns. Although they are assisted by decongestants, expectorants, antitussives, analgesics, moisture, irrigation, and cortisone nasal sprays, antibiotics and surgery still remain the foundation for treating America's most common chronic disease. Yet if this approach had a high rate of cure, we would probably not be experiencing an epidemic in which nearly one out of every seven Americans now suffers from a chronic sinus condition.

Although medical science has created ever stronger antibiotics and developed ever more effective surgical techniques, we seem to be winning battles but losing the war against sinus disease. Otolaryngologists (ear, nose, and throat specialists) are the professionals usually assigned the task of treating the most challenging chronic sinus sufferers—the first group of people with chronic sinusitis described in Chapter 3. The sinus patients in this group suffer the most discomfort. Before arriving at the specialist's office, they might have been fighting a sinus infection for several months to a year, and in many cases, two or three years. Most of them have already been through several courses of antibiotics without success. Their physicians have given up; these patients are considered treatment failures.

The initial evaluation by the ENT doctor usually includes the application of a topical decongestant in the nose and a nasal bacterial culture, followed by a physical examination of the nose, throat, and sinuses. The specimen for the culture needs to be obtained right from the opening of the sinus ducts (ostia) or else it will be of little value. The ENT specialist is attempting to identify the specific bacteria that are infecting the sinuses. The bacteria found in the nose are not usually the same as those infecting the sinuses. The culture should be performed by someone who has had a lot of experience in locating the ostia (usually an ENT specialist), so that the results will be a true reflection of the bacteria that are actually causing the infection. This test is critical to the selection of the most effective antibiotic. As a result of the more accurate performance of this test, many specialists have seen a dramatic increase in *Staphylococcus aureus* in the sinuses. This is one of the most difficult bacteria to treat.

Subsequent diagnostic procedures might include a sinus CT scan to determine if, after a course of an antibiotic, there are any lingering pockets of infection; rhinoscopy, the insertion of a flexible "telescope" into the nasal passages to see if there is any obstruction around the ostia (this procedure is probably performed more often by allergists); a nasal cytogram, a microscopic inspection of cells from the nasal mucous membrane; and a complete battery of skin and/or blood tests to identify possible allergies.

The initial treatment usually includes a ten-day to two-week course of one of the stronger antibiotics—Cipro, Ceftin, or Suprax (the latter, however, is not effective for *Staphylococ-*

cus)—in addition to the treatment regimen described in Chapter 4, with particular emphasis on irrigation. If this fails—meaning either that there is no improvement or that the infection is still present on the CT scan or recurs shortly after the antibiotic is stopped—further evaluation using one or more of the diagnostic procedures previously mentioned will be necessary. Depending on the results, either a different antibiotic or surgery will be offered.

Sinus surgery has improved dramatically in the past three years. If there is an obstruction of the ostio-meatal complex (the opening of the sinus duct into the nasal passage), surgery is usually recommended. The endoscope, another type of flexible "telescope," has taken sinus surgery to an even higher level of success. The most common endoscopic sinus surgery is a bilateral middle antrostomy, in which the maxillary sinus ostia are enlarged from 2 millimeters to about 10 or 12 millimeters (approximately the width of a dime). This procedure is a marked improvement over the surgery that created naso-antral windows. The opening of a naso-antral window was about the same size as the opening created by an antrostomy, but it went entirely through the bony medial wall (nasal side) of the maxillary sinus. The new procedure is not only less destructive, but preserves the normal direction of mucus flow in the sinus. Mucus naturally flows out through the sinus duct and into the nose. The fact that the naso-antral window was not in the best position to enhance drainage greatly diminished its rate of success, despite the large opening it produced. Many patients who have had this surgery, or the Caldwell-Luc operation or ethmoidectomy (other surgical procedures not performed as often anymore), continue to have sinus problems and not infrequently require additional surgery. So far, endoscopic surgery looks good; it is performed on an outpatient basis under local anesthesia, and patients can expect to miss only about one week of work. However, it is certainly not inexpensive. Surgeons will charge from $4,000 to $10,000 for the procedure. Following surgery, patients are often instructed to use Nasalcrom or one of the cortisone sprays for several months. Since it has been widely performed for only about three years, long-term success rates for endoscopic surgery are not yet available. However, it is clearly an improvement over the previous procedures.

Sinus surgery has been and probably will continue to be most successful in those instances in which it eliminates one of the obstructive causes of sinusitis, such as a deviated septum, an enlarged or distorted nasal turbinate (turbinate hypertrophy), cysts, or polyps. In these cases the surgery eliminates causes, but where there is no obstruction the surgery will only be treating symptoms and the underlying factors that created the chronic sinusitis will still be present afterward. This is precisely why chronic sinusitis is usually considered an incurable condition. Whether the chronic sinus sufferer has repeated debilitating infections over several years, a mild infection with fatigue over most of a lifetime, or a persistent inflammation resulting in congestion, headaches, postnasal drip, and a weakened sense of smell and taste, for the most part, traditional medicine offers only symptomatic treatment and the prognosis, "You're going to have to learn to live with it."

7 HOLISTIC MEDICINE: INTRODUCTION

If you would rather not learn to live with your condition and a diminished quality of life, I would like to take you on a journey into an exciting new frontier of medicine. For the past five years I have been using the holistic option for treating chronic sinusitis. Commitment to this approach results in a 100 percent success rate in either significantly improving or curing the condition. The holistic approach is *not* an alternative to traditional medicine but a complement to it. In confronting a chronic disease such as sinusitis, why not choose a treatment program that incorporates many therapeutic modalities, not merely those sanctioned by medical science? I believe that all of the techniques described in Part II will eventually be validated by the scientific community. Meanwhile, I will attest to their remarkable efficacy while continuing to refine them.

Holistic medicine is a unique blend of health education and medical treatment. Practitioners of this approach regard health as a state of balance and wholeness. The word *health* is related to the Anglo-Saxon word *haelen*, meaning "to make whole." The benefits of the holistic approach include a heightened sense of physical, mental, emotional, spiritual, and social well-being. Holistic medicine encompasses elements of many types of medicine, including allopathic (whose practitioners are M.D.'s), osteopathic (D.O.'s), chiropractic (D.C.'s), naturopathic (N.D.'s), Chinese (O.M.D.'s), environmental, and preventive. It is based in part on the relatively new science of psychoneuroimmunology.

The word *doctor* derives from a Latin word meaning "teacher." The holistic doctor works in partnership with patients to guide them through their own process of self-healing. Rather than being a fixer of the broken part of the body, a holistic physician becomes a teacher of health, enabling patients to repair themselves and to take better care of their body, mind, emotions, spirit, and relationships. Physician-philosopher Hippocrates' admonition "Physician, heal thyself"—still taught to medical students 2,400 years after the words were first spoken—was an invitation to the physician to discover the power of the healing process in the only way it can be discovered: through personal experience. Hippocrates was saying that if physicians are to become effective health educators, the best way to teach is to practice what you preach.

This approach is directed toward treating causes rather than symptoms. Unfortunately, it does not often lend itself to the "quick fix" to which our society has become so accustomed. Whether our need is for food, energy, entertainment, transportation, communication, or health care, we look to satisfy it in the fastest, simplest, and easiest way. Science and technology have attempted to keep pace with these desires, and indeed, they have performed incredible, at times almost miraculous, feats that have allowed an ease of living never before experienced in human history. However, there is a price to be paid for all of this comfort. Technology is helping us to destroy our environment—to pollute our air, poison our food and water, deplete our soil, thin our protective ozone layer, decimate our forests at the rate of one acre every second, and cause the extinction of nearly one hundred species of plants and animals daily! Our own species, *Homo sapiens*, might not be far behind.

Sinus disease might be the proverbial canary in the coal mine. There is already evidence that its prevalence will soon be followed by higher rates of every one of the most common varieties of lung disease and most forms of cancers. In the past forty years, lung cancer has increased more than any other form of cancer in the United States. The mortality rate of asthma, the most common chronic childhood disease, has more than doubled in the past ten years. The incidence of chronic bronchitis and emphysema, along with asthma, have all increased by 50 percent during the past decade (1981–1991). Physicians are now witnessing in their own examination rooms the magnitude of the health hazards of air pollution.

To treat these conditions most effectively, a twofold approach is necessary: minimizing and, if possible, eliminating the harmful environmental factors that have contributed to the condition, and then strengthening the body and its natural defense mechanism, the immune system. Chapter 8 will focus on creating a healthy environment; Chapters 9 through 14 will explore the various aspects of internal treatment.

8 How to Help Your Sinuses by Changing Your Environment

Over the past three years I have met with air filtration, humidification, negative ionization, and indoor air pollution experts; allergists; specialists in environmental medicine; and ecological architects. With their guidance and their state-of-the-art technology, I have learned a great deal about environmental health. The information in this chapter is a result of that education.

There is nothing more important to human health and survival than the air we breathe. The sinuses and the nose, our first line of defense against unhealthy air, are a sensitive gauge of air quality. Ideal quality is rated by clarity (freedom from pollutants), humidity (between 40 and 60 percent), temperature (between 65° and 85°F), oxygen content (21 percent of total volume and 100 percent saturation), and negative ion content (3,000 to 6,000 .001-micron ions per cubic centimeter). Air that is clean, moist, warm, oxygen rich, and high in negative ions is the healthiest air a human being can breathe.

Not only are we dependent on oxygen for survival, but every part of the human body thrives with a maximum supply of oxygen. If your respiratory tract is defective because of a nasal, sinus, or lung ailment, or if the amount of oxygen available in the air is relatively low (for example, air high in carbon monoxide, air at higher altitudes, or stale indoor air), your body is receiving less than its optimal requirement of oxygen.

Negative ions are electrically charged particles that vitalize or freshen the air. Studies have shown that they can help to create a feeling of well-being while reducing pain, healing burns, suppressing bacterial growth, stimulating plant growth, and improving the sweeping motion of the cilia on the mucous membrane. The highest concentrations of negative ions, in some places as high as 40,000 ions per cubic centimeter, have been found on mountaintops, along seacoasts, near rushing streams and waterfalls, and in pine forests (pine needles and the pointed leaves of other plants cause negative ions to be generated in the surrounding air). Many who have spent time in these environments have described feeling very good or at least experiencing an improvement in their sense of well-being, and although there are certainly other factors involved, negative ions contribute significantly to the experience.

The majority of Americans spend 90 percent of their time indoors, where, the EPA says, the air can be as much as 100 times more polluted than outdoor air. The average negative ion content in indoor air is 200 ions per cubic centimeter. Few of us live in clean, moist environments that are warm year-round; even fewer live in the mountains, on a beach, or in the woods. For the 34 million people whose sinuses are already feeling the pain that comes from breathing unhealthy air, and for anyone else who wants to enjoy optimum health, here are some ways to minimize the risks of breathing poor-quality air and to prevent sinus disease.

LOCATION

Where we live, work, play, or otherwise spend our time is critical to our health. If you are considering a move and need help in evaluating a potential location, use this list from Richard L. Crowther's book *Indoor Air: Risks and Remedies*:

- Locate in houses and buildings that minimize the impact of outdoor air pollution.
- Locate in a city, town, or county that has minimal air pollution.
- Locate on a hill rather than in a valley, where pollution is more apt to concentrate.
- Do not locate near a major highway or traffic intersection.
- Do not locate next to a parking lot.
- Do not locate downwind from a power plant, chemical plant, or processing plant.
- Do not locate near industrial operations.
- Do not locate near businesses that emit pollutants.
- Do not locate near a railroad line that carries hazardous materials.
- Do not locate near airfields.
- Do not locate on land farmed with pesticides and chemical fertilizers.
- Locate away from agricultural fields that are sprayed.
- Do not live under or near high-voltage power lines.
- Locate away from stagnant waterways.
- Locate out of the air pollution or "seepage" range of oil or gas wells.
- Locate a safe distance from any mining operations.
- Locate close to a park, near a forest, or within a natural setting.
- Locate in a small, healthful rural or seacoast community.
- Consider the effect of altitude on air quality.
- Consider prevailing daily and seasonal wind patterns.
- Before moving to a city, review an air quality record of the past several years.

- In urban or rural locations, consider sites for passive solar orientation and exposure.
- South-sloping sites are preferable for drainage and solar advantage.
- Avoid being in a "shadow path" during winter months in a cold climate.
- Avoid sites with high levels of radon or radioactivity.
- Before buying a property, get soils, radon, and water tests (if a well is planned).
- Check municipal water quality.

In addition, if allergies are a problem for you, it would be helpful to check with the local allergy society on the predominant allergens in that area. I would also suggest living there for at least one month before making the commitment to move.

It is unlikely that all of these locational criteria can be met, but they can provide a basis for a thorough evaluation. If you are going to relocate and have the freedom to choose, avoid the following regions: Southern California, the Northeast, and the Texas Gulf Coast. The healthiest air can be found along the West Coast (with the distinct exception of the Los Angeles metropolitan area and southward) and anywhere in Hawaii other than Honolulu.

ECOLOGICAL ARCHITECTURE

If you are contemplating the construction of a new home, the concept of ecological architecture could help considerably in creating a healthy environment. *Ecology* is defined in Webster's *New World Dictionary* as "the branch of biology that deals with the relationship between living organisms and their environment." Used as a modifier for the word *architecture*, it simply means the design of a dwelling that is sensitive to human health and gentle to the earth. Once we have considered the microclimate and the site, our biologic needs, behavior patterns, and, most important, our budgetary limitations, nature will then dictate the design. Self-sufficiency through use of sun, air, earth, and water for heating, cooling, ventilation, and even electrical power is a realistic goal of an ecological design.

Common objectives regarding construction methods and materials include

- avoiding the use of plastic or other materials made of toxic ingredients that harmfully outgas in the indoor environment;
- the use of nontoxic natural materials in preference to synthetic materials;
- design concern for sensitivities, allergies, or chronic health problems;
- concern that nature's ecologic sustainability and well-being should not be diminished by what is built; and
- a responsibility to conceive, design, build, and furnish a home or building to a "healthy home" ecologic ethic.

This is a holistic approach emphasizing the ecological bond between site and architecture. Preservation and wise use of our planet's resources in construction and throughout the lifetime of a home is fundamental to ecological design. For the sinus sufferer, a home must be clean, moist, warm, and oxygen and negative ion rich. The fact that it is designed in harmony with the atmosphere and the earth makes this a totally integrated concept.

I fully appreciate that most readers of this book will neither move nor design their own home as a result of what they read here. However, I want to present as many environmental treatment options as possible. Each can have a profound impact on your state of health and ultimately your quality of life.

HEALTHY HOMES

You can create an oasis of healthy indoor air in your own home. In the desert an oasis provides water. In the sea of hazardous air in which we live, a healthy home or business can provide an oasis in which to breathe life-enhancing air.

Solving the problem of indoor air pollution entails both treatment and prevention. Treatment involves accepting pollutants as inevitable components of indoor air and attempting to reduce them as much as possible with air cleaners, furnace filters, negative ion generators, ventilation, air duct cleaning, and carpet cleaning. Prevention is an attempt to eliminate the sources of the pollutants, especially those to which you might be most sensitive.

AIR CLEANERS AND NEGATIVE ION GENERATORS

As many as one million hospital admissions a year are attributed to poor indoor air quality. In recent years, as the EPA and private health organizations have publicized the problem of indoor air pollution, we have seen a proliferation of several hundred types of air cleaners, almost as many as there are indoor air pollutants. According to Michael Berry, Ph.D., manager of the EPA's Indoor Air Project, the most potentially harmful pollutants are radon and the "biologicals," including pollen, mold, plant spores, dust mites, bacteria, and viruses. The pollutants most harmful to the respiratory tract are less than one micron in size. Regardless of their origin, size, or health-damaging effects, air pollutants can be described as free-floating particles in the air. Figure 6 shows the specific size ranges of the most common pollutants. The unit of measurement used for tiny air particles is the micron. An average hair strand is 100 microns thick, and about 400 1-micron par-

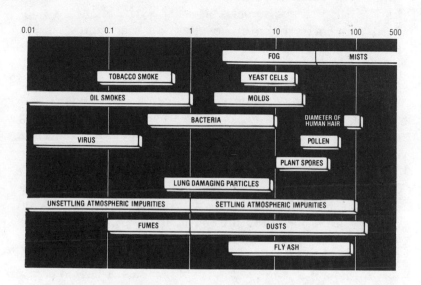

FIGURE 6   *Relative Size of Common Air Contaminants*

ticles would fit into the dot over the "i" in the word *micron*. The primary job of air cleaners is to remove as many of these particles as possible, the biologicals as well as the combustion products, particulates, chemicals, fumes, and odors (see Table 1, p. 17–18. Radon, if present, requires the sealing of basement cracks and improvement of basement ventilation. Air cleaners do not remove radon from the air.

The strategy for solving the problem of indoor air pollution involves air cleaning and improved ventilation. Air cleaning devices can include furnace filters, portable stand-alone units, and negative ion generators. The efficiency of air cleaners is evaluated by their ability to filter a certain percentage of a certain size of pollutant. The HEPA filter (an acronym for high efficiency particulate arrestor) removes 95 percent of all 0.3 micron particulates and larger. This includes pollen, plant spores, most animal dander, dust, wood, and tobacco smoke, fumes, bacteria, and some viruses. This type of filter is standard equipment for most hospital operating suites, and is found in many of the more expensive free-standing air cleaners and furnace filters. It requires a strong fan or a booster fan to move air through it due to its increased efficiency.

Negative ion generators have the capacity to remove particles as small as .001 micron. This would include all viruses, dust, and outdoor air pollutants. Negative ion generator units are presently available in a variety of shapes, sizes, and prices. Their primary liability is that since the negatively charged particles are free in the air, they will attach to the nearest grounding surface. This means that dirty residues will accumulate on metal objects, including unseen nails used in dry-wall construction. This problem can be minimized by placing the ionizer at least two feet away from any wall or ceiling surface.

Although it is not yet available for sale, I have recently learned about a free-standing air cleaner using new technology with both HEPA filtration and negative ions. Its filter is 99 percent effective in removing all particles 0.2 micron and larger in a room of 300 square feet. It is capable of cleaning larger rooms at the same efficiency but at a slower rate. This not only cleans the air more efficiently than a standard HEPA filter, but also provides the healthy biological effects of negative ions.

Electrostatic air cleaners (both central and free-standing) produce positive ions as they filter the air. On their first day of operation they are 85 percent efficient on all 1-micron particles and larger, but in order to maintain that efficiency they require cleaning every two weeks. For most of us, this makes them impractical and inconvenient. They also produce ozone, which, as discussed in Chapter 2, can be a potential health hazard.

AIR DUCT CLEANING

A company called Monster Vac recently cleaned—for the first time ever—my home's entire air duct system. I was amazed by what emanated from the ducts of this thirteen-year-old house after two hours of high-intensity vacuuming. I thought to myself, "It's no wonder I suffered with sinus problems for so long!" If the air ducts are filthy, it is nearly impossible for your furnace filter to clean the air in your home. After the air is filtered, it still has to travel through the ducts before you breathe it. I recommend air duct cleaning as part of the environmental treatment program. Depending on the size of your home, the cost could be between $200 and $250. To find this type of company in your city, look in the Yellow Pages under "Furnaces, Cleaning and Repairing."

CARPET CLEANING

Carpets are one of the most common sources of indoor air pollutants. They are excellent traps and hold onto dust, pollen, and microorganisms. While this helps to keep those particles out of the breathing zone, their gradual accumulation can become great enough to create a sustainable culture of bacteria, yeast, and mold. In fact, many allergists recommend that their patients dispose of all their carpets.

While it is true that carpets harbor pollutants, it is possible to keep them clean. This poses a challenge to the homemaker. Conventional vacuum cleaners are designed to remove and retain the visible dirt, which means particles greater than 10 microns. Most of the particles and microorganisms that are too small to be seen are also smaller than the pores in the vacuum cleaner bag. This allows most of them to blow through the bag and into the room, settling back onto the carpets and furniture. If a forced-air heating system is running, the airborne particles can be drawn into the air ducts, contributing to their contamination as well. Also, as the bag fills, airflow decreases, causing uneven cleaning.

To prevent these problems I suggest a vacuum cleaner that uses either a HEPA-type filter or water-capture. Either one removes even sub-visible dust and bacteria from the air. The water-capture types also have a continuously maximum airflow because they won't clog like a bag or filter. Both of these vacuums are expensive, costing in the vicinity of $1,000.

Many people have their carpets professionally cleaned. However, due to their chemical composition, the most common cleaning agents are often worse than having dirty carpets. Alcohols, petroleum distillates, ammonia, dry-cleaning substances, and scents often cause headaches, mental "fuzziness," lethargy, and a general feeling of discomfort. Cleaning-agent residues may often cause respiratory irritation.

Before contracting with a carpet cleaner, check his references and insist on a non-scented cleaning agent that uses no petroleum distillates, alcohol, ammonia, dry-cleaning–type chemicals or enzymes, and has no suds that can be left in the carpet. Check his work to be sure he leaves no damp areas. This ensures maximum removal of all agents and enhances drying time. If the carpet stays wet for several days, bacteria and molds can grow rapidly.

VENTILATION, OXYGEN, AND PLANTS

All indoor spaces, whether residential, commercial, industrial, or recreational, require some type of ventilation to provide breathable air for occupants, to furnish combustion air for cooking and heating, and to remove stale air filled with toxins and particulates. Commercial buildings are required by code to have even more efficient ventilation systems than residences. The American Society of Heating, Refrigerating and Air-Conditioning Engineers (ASHRAE) says that air should be replaced at the rate of 15 cubic feet per minute per person, but most systems fall below this minimum standard.

Improving ventilation will help relieve indoor air pollution as long as the outdoor air isn't dirtier than the air it is replacing. Local pollution sources, such as fumes from toxic waste leakage, wood burning, a neighboring industrial plant, a heavily trafficked highway, or crop spraying can render outdoor air unacceptable for indoor ventilation. Several days a year, Los Angeles residents are advised to keep all windows and doors closed and ventilation ducts shut to prevent the heavily polluted outdoor air from entering homes and businesses. In areas like this, it becomes a challenge to balance the health benefit of highly oxygenated outdoor air and the liability of the pollutants that come with it. Outdoor aerobic exercise presents a similar dilemma. If you live in a heavily polluted environment, I recommend exercising outside and ventilating your home and office well when outdoor air is good, but exercise indoors and keep windows and doors closed during periods of heavy pollution.

Air-conditioning systems are a helpful means of ventilation for people with respiratory and allergy problems. These systems remove excess moisture from the air, lowering its temperature. In less humid conditions there is a reduction of molds and spores, and with the windows closed there is also a marked decrease in pollen from the outdoors.

Natural cross-ventilation is effective in reducing indoor air pollution if the placement of the intake vents is low and the outlets for the flow-through air high. Operable windows on commercial buildings and a good location for the outdoor air intake—away from garage entrances or loading docks—are also important factors in improving indoor air quality. Mechanical ventilation with exhaust fans can certainly help in removing indoor pollutants, but such fans are most efficient when used in a confined space. Private offices or single-occupant rooms where smoking, cooking, and other fume-producing activities take place are ideal environments for mechanical ventilation.

Rooms producing commercial toxic or odoriferous fumes; spaces subject to bacterial and viral contamination, such as rest rooms; and indoor areas that present specific respiratory hazards all need optimized ventilation. Mold is a special problem in moist conditions. Adequate ventilation along with sunshine can help to reduce moisture and subsequently suppress mold.

The technology of ventilation can be complex, but the basic principle of displacing interior air with outdoor air and increasing the rate of fresh air flow is critical to treating the problem of indoor air pollution. Besides natural cross-ventilation and exhaust fans, other devices used to enhance ventilation and indoor air quality are air-to-air heat exchangers, makeup air units, attic fans, vortex fans, and ceiling fans. Remember that even if the "fresh" air is filthy, an effective air cleaner combined with good ventilation is still a winning combination.

Adequate ventilation not only helps reduce indoor air pollution, but is the primary source of indoor oxygen. Plants can offer an esthetically pleasant secondary source. Although the oxygen output from indoor plants is not great, plants with large leaf surfaces that grow rapidly are capable of enhancing air quality. Attached greenhouses and atria filled with plants that effectively absorb carbon dioxide and oxygenate the air (spider plants do this very well) can improve the indoor environment while humidifying the air.

In recent years, studies conducted at the John Stennis Space Center in Mississippi have shown that plants can also act as effective filters. Researchers estimate that in the average home, fifteen spider plants could remove the formaldehyde emissions from furniture, walls, and cooking. Aloe vera, philodendron, pothus, draceana, ficus, English ivy, and chrysanthemums were found to reduce levels of formaldehyde, benzene, trichloroethylene, and carbon dioxide.

Plants can help improve indoor air as oxygenators, filters, and humidifiers.

PREVENTION

Prevention of indoor air pollution involves eliminating pollutants at the source. Doctors who specialize in environmental medicine and some allergists can do skin and blood tests to help you identify pollutants to which you are particularly sensitive or allergic. These doctors are not always easy to find, nor are the tests always definitive, but they can help. With the use of environmentally sensitive architectural principles, a healthier home can be created. A major preventive strategy is the use of interior materials that emit no pollutants. Natural products such as wood, cotton, and metals are preferable to the lower-cost synthetic materials such as fiberboard, polyester, and plastics.

Choosing to forgo a fireplace or wood-burning stove would be helpful, as would using a high-efficiency furnace with a sealed combustion unit to vent exhaust gases to the outside. Switch to nontoxic cleaning substances, including ordinary soap, vinegar, zephiran, and Air Therapy (you can find a listing of such cleaners in *Nontoxic, Natural, & Earthwise* by Debra Lynn Dadd). Smoking should be relegated to the outdoors or to a well-ventilated enclosed space. If radon levels exceed the acceptable ASHRAE standard, radon control measures should be implemented. Formaldehyde from insulation can be eliminated by using the substitutes of cellulose and fiberglass insulation.

HUMIDIFICATION

Optimum indoor air quality requires air containing between 40 and 60 percent relative humidity. Moisture provided by room humidifiers can benefit sinus sufferers. These humidifiers are helpful in the winter (heavy "sinus season" runs from November through March), even in humid, cold-weather climates, because most heating systems dry the indoor air considerably.

Central humidifiers, those that attach to the furnace, are more convenient but do not humidify an individual room as well as a portable humidifier can when the door to the room is closed. The major problem with central humidifiers is that most of them are the reservoir type, with a tray of standing water that breeds mold and bacteria. I recommend the flow-through type of central humidifier, e.g. Aprilaire or General, which eliminates the stagnant water problem and is easy to maintain. Depending on the model, size of your home, and installation, this humidifier would probably cost about $300.

Humidifiers are not the only option for moisturizing your home. The installation of waterfalls, indoor spas, and swimming pools will all add a lot of moisture to the house, but, of course, they are expensive to install and maintain. It might surprise you to learn that even the moisture from human breath and sweat, along with that from cooking, baths, showers, and plants, adds significantly to a home's humidity.

9 HOW TO HELP YOUR SINUSES BY CHANGING YOURSELF

The immune system is that wondrous component of the human body that protects us from disease. It includes the bone marrow, spleen, liver, lymph nodes, and white blood cells. The study of this field, immunology, is still, relatively speaking, in its infancy. Physicians have known empirically for a long time that if an individual has an ample supply of oxygen, eats a well-balanced diet, drinks enough liquids, and gets enough sleep, he or she should be healthy. The fact that so many of us comply with these basic requirements but get sick anyway has prompted researchers to ask the following: Is all air healthy, and if not, what is healthy air? What does a well-balanced, healthy diet consist of? What are the best liquids to drink and how much should we drink? How much sleep do we require? And, most important, What other factors can weaken or strengthen the immune system? The first question, regarding air quality, I have already answered. In the remainder of this text I will attempt to answer the other questions and to provide a glimpse of the exciting new science of psychoneuroimmunology (PNI).

Medical science is able to cure only about 25 percent of

all disease. Nevertheless, traditional medicine is for the most part disease oriented. Its focus is on fixing the broken or malfunctioning part of the body about which the patient complains most. This approach is extremely effective in treating acute illness and medical and surgical emergencies. About 75 percent of the time, however, successful medical treatment simply means that symptoms are (1) alleviated until the body's natural healing mechanism and immune system can finish the job, as with colds, sore throats, and most viral infections; (2) relieved and controlled with long-term medication, surgery, diet, and other measures, as in chronic sinusitis, arthritis, diabetes, high blood pressure, and allergies; or (3) variably relieved with drugs and surgery, as in many forms of cancer; Parkinson's, Alzheimer's, and other neurologic diseases; and AIDS.

As medicine begins its shift from a disease- to a health-oriented approach, the opportunities for curing chronic disease have increased tremendously. Herbert Benson, M.D., director of the Mind/Body Clinic in the Department of Behavioral Medicine at the Harvard University School of Medicine, has shown how relaxation techniques can treat high blood pressure, migraine headaches, and many other common and chronic ailments. He has also documented the healing power of prayer, which I address again in Chapter 13. Bernie Siegel, M.D., of the Yale University School of Medicine, a past president of the American Holistic Medical Association (AHMA) and the author of the best-seller *Love, Medicine and Miracles,* has had extraordinary results in treating his cancer patients with holistic medicine. C. Norman Shealy, M.D., a neurosurgeon and the cofounder and original president of the AHMA, has seen remarkable results for more than fifteen years in the holistic treatment of chronic pain. Using a holistic approach, Dean Ornish, M.D., at the University of California School of Medicine at San Francisco, has been able to *reverse* coronary artery disease (the leading cause of death in the

United States) in his patients—something that has never before been demonstrated. He describes this method in his book *Dr. Dean Ornish's Program for Reversing Heart Disease.*

If holistic medicine has been shown as effective in treating migraine headaches, high blood pressure, chronic pain, cancer, and heart disease, surely it also can be used to treat the nation's most common chronic disease: chronic sinusitis. In fact, the sinuses respond quite well to holistic treatment. The following pages give a brief description of my approach to holistic health and the internal treatment of chronic sinusitis. Each component warrants an entire book, and, indeed, makes reference to several relevant works. The program I present here is one I have taught for the past five years in the treatment of sinus disease and other chronic conditions. Its focus is on learning to experience greater health and well-being in body, mind, emotions, spirit, and relationships. As by-products of this course of study and of treating the whole person, not only do sinuses feel better, but patients feel a greater sense of vitality and enjoyment of life than they have experienced before.

Learning to become your own healer requires a commitment to loving yourself, a willingness to change, an open mind, time, effort, and patience. You can choose to do as much or as little as feels comfortable to you. Many of my patients have experienced great relief from their sinus symptoms after working on just the physical component. However, if you are interested in curing sinus disease, you must go further. Trust your intuition and remember that, as the "physician" directing this program, you are following an inexact prescription, therefore, you can't make mistakes.

Physical fitness is the first of five aspects of holistic health that will be discussed. None of the others seems to be as easy or quick to change as the physical (and believe me, I've tried). Yet the cure for chronic sinusitis and any other chronic disease lies in healing not only the physical but the less tangible parts of ourselves: the mind, emotions, spirit, and relationships. All of these aspects of health lie beyond the scope of our five senses.

The nonphysical aspect of my practice is based on psychoneuroimmunology, the complicated interplay between the body and the mind, which derives its name from *psycho*, the brain, *neuro*, the nervous system, and *immunology*, the study of the immune system. This is the scientific basis of holistic medicine. It has also been called mind-body medicine or behavioral medicine. Research has confirmed that our thoughts, beliefs, attitudes, emotions, and relationships (both with other people and with a higher power) can either strengthen or weaken our immune system. This process occurs in the transmission of messenger molecules (neuropeptides) through the nervous system to be received by the immune system. In the practice of mind-body medicine, the mind aspect encompasses mental, emotional, spiritual, and social health. The condition referred to as stress or emotional stress can result from an imbalance in any or all of these four aspects of health. A critical factor in the cause of chronic sinusitis and all other disease is this hidden, largely unconscious part of ourselves.

As I practice medicine, I see myself as a teacher. The course of study I teach is holistic health. Many of my "students" (patients) come to "class" monthly for an extended consultation. Initially they come for the treatment of a chronic disease or with the desire to experience a greater degree of health. The majority of these students are chronic sinus sufferers.

My "curriculum" has evolved over the past five years. It was designed to implement the principles of mind-body medicine and to help others practice holistic medicine on themselves, as I am doing on myself. There is no doubt that each of us has the potential to become our own best healer. In order to assume greater responsibility for our own health, however, we first need to educate ourselves.

What follows is a set of healthy options from which to

choose. Using your intuition to refine and personalize this process of self-healing, you will experience a greater degree of
physical fitness, vigor and vitality, peace of mind, ability to use
your gifts, awareness of and ability to express feelings, connectedness with others and with a higher power, and very
healthy sinuses. You will become more aware of what feels
good and what doesn't, and you will learn to make choices that
are life enhancing. You are, in essence, learning to love yourself, and in so doing will be better able to love others. This is
a program based on the belief that love is our most powerful
healer. Each of us is the best person to administer that medicine to ourselves. It is an inexpensive drug without unpleasant
side effects, and one on which you cannot overdose.

Chapters 10 through 14 provide a prescription for improving the five components of human health. I have referred
to several books for those who would like to explore these areas
in greater depth. I have tried to simplify each component and
have suggested "exercises" to help you find your own path to
a greater level of physical, mental, emotional, spiritual, and
social fitness. These exercises must be practiced regularly in
order to be effective. (However, if a particular exercise does
not feel comfortable to you, don't do it.) If you are willing to
wait—and remember, it took years for you to develop your
current state of health—I promise you not only that they will
all work, but that every one of them will feel good. Keep in
mind that although this is a course with a lot of homework,
there are no grades, so enjoy yourself!

10 PHYSICAL HEALTH

After almost twenty years as a physician it has become clear to me that for anyone experiencing physical discomfort, life is not much fun. In order to begin work on the other aspects of health, including mental and spiritual, it helps to have some degree of physical stability and symptom relief.

The holistic approach to physical fitness helps patients become more aware of and develop greater respect and appreciation for their bodies. Through this process you will gain a much greater sensitivity to your own body and learn how it functions optimally.

SINUS TREATMENT

Because the majority of you have sinus problems, it is important to begin with an aggressive approach to treating your sinusitis. The same holds true when you deal with any chronic condition. Make sure that you have consulted with your physician and have made an attempt to treat your ailment with the best methods that traditional medicine has to offer, even if they only provide symptomatic relief.

For sinus sufferers this would mean using most of what I have already recommended, including antibiotics, decongestants, expectorants, analgesics, irrigation, saline sprays, pure drinking water, an air cleaner, a humidifier, a negative ion generator, air duct cleaning, and plants. All of these will make a significant improvement in your condition.

Another option I use with chronic sinus patients who have tried numerous courses of antibiotics without success is to treat for systemic yeast infections. Repeated antibiotics can make you much more susceptible to yeast. Yeast (*Candida albicans*) is an opportunistic fungus that is present but doesn't cause infection until the immune system has been adversely affected. Most commonly it causes vaginal infections in women. Quite often it follows a course of an antibiotic. In fact, yeast infections are much more common in women. Both yeast and antibiotics have been shown to depress immune function, thereby contributing to chronic sinus infections. Yeast infections seem to be much more prevalent than was previously assumed. Two excellent books on this subject are *The Yeast Connection: A Medical Breakthrough* by William G. Crook, M.D., and the recently released *The Yeast Syndrome* by John Parks Trowbridge, M.D., and Morton Walker, D.P.M.

Systemic, or whole-body, yeast infections are not easily detected. If the more common antibiotics are not doing the job for your sinus infection, you might suggest to your doctor that you try a course of Nizoral, a prescription antiyeast antibiotic. It should be taken daily for one month, and then every second or third day for the next month. It can be toxic to the liver, however; therefore, a liver blood test is recommended before starting, and again after one month of treatment. Neither Nystatin, also a prescription drug, nor Cantrol, an over-the-counter alternative that can be found in most health-food stores, are quite as effective as Nizoral.

The standard antiyeast diet initially includes protein, vegetables, and limited amounts of carbohydrates. It is best to eliminate completely the following foods during the first two to three weeks of antiyeast treatments: fruits and fruit juices, breads, milk products, cheese, yogurt, sugar, fried foods, sausage, hot dogs, fermented foods (i.e., all alcohol products, vinegar, and pickled foods), leavened and baked goods, mushrooms, and vitamins made with a yeast base. In rare cases you may need to also exclude grains entirely if they aggravate your symptoms. Beans, grains, and protein foods should be rotated to prevent the aggravation of possible food allergies. Rotation means not repeating the same food in a four-day cycle. At the end of three weeks, add one new fruit to your diet each day. Pears and bananas seem to be best tolerated. "Listen" to your body and note if your symptoms get worse.

The overall antiyeast food rotation plan is usually maintained for three months to one year. You must stay consistent for this time frame in order to obtain long-term benefits. The diet should be personalized to best fit your needs by a nutritionally oriented physician, nutritionist, or a naturopathic physician.

Acidophilus is also suggested as part of an effective antiyeast program. This beneficial bowel bacteria serves as a first line of defense against a multitude of pathogens, inhibits yeast overgrowth, assists in the absorption of nutrients in the small bowel, and produces B-vitamins. I recommend either Ethical Nutrients Maxidophilus in a powder, or Nature's Way Primadophilus in a tablet. Depending upon which one you choose, take either two tablets two times per day, or one-quarter to one-half teaspoon two times per day with water at least one-half hour before meals.

An effective alternative to acidophilus for the first three months of an antiyeast program is Flora Balance. Available in most health-food stores, the naturally occurring bacteria laterosporos quickly reduces the candida overgrowth.

DIET

"We are what we eat." I have heard that saying many times, but it never made much of an impact until I began changing my diet in the process of treating my own chronic sinusitis. I am now convinced that most chronic medical conditions can be helped significantly by a healthy diet. With specific regard to the sinuses, the change I recommend most is to avoid milk and dairy products. They tend to increase and thicken mucus secretions. If you would like to compensate for the loss of calcium in your own or your child's diet, the following foods are especially rich in calcium: broccoli, kale, sesame seeds and sesame seed butter, tofu, sea vegetables, and soy cheese. You can also buy a liquid calcium and magnesium combination at most health-food stores. An adequate daily dose for an adult female is 1,200 mg of calcium and 500 to 600 mg of magnesium.

Sugar should also be avoided, especially if you suspect that yeast is contributing to your sinusitis. A nutritionist once asked me, "Would you fill the gas tank of your car with sand?" She felt that filling your body with sugar is equally destructive. Sugar not only has no nutritional value, it is also harmful.

Caffeine is a drug to which most Americans are addicted. It is a stimulant that races our engines for a few hours, only to leave us with a greater sense of fatigue when the effect wears off. The quick fix for this state of low energy is usually to drink another cup of coffee or tea or another bottle of caffeine-rich soda pop. Your entire body suffers as a result of being on a perpetual "roller coaster." The best way to break this addiction is to do it very gradually, substituting noncaffeinated beverages such as herb tea or a roasted-grain beverage. Be aware of the possible withdrawal symptoms of headache, fatigue, and irritability.

I'm sure that most of you are familiar with the recommendation to decrease your consumption of red meat and egg yolks. Both are significant sources of cholesterol, which is a major contributor to heart disease. Recent research by the USDA suggests that a low-fat diet may also strengthen your immune system. Alcohol should be consumed only in moderate amounts (two to three beers, or one cocktail, or a glass of wine per day). Studies have shown that complete abstainers from alcohol have a slightly shorter life expectancy than those who drink in moderate amounts. However, if a yeast infection is aggravating your chronic sinusitis, don't drink any alcohol for at least three months during treatment. Since sugar and alcohol seem to be major dietary contributors to the problem of yeast, it is not difficult to understand how the typical American diet has encouraged this widespread infection.

Try to decrease your consumption of food additives. These include chemical preservatives (such as BHA, BHT, sodium nitrite, and sulfites), artificial colors, and artificial sweeteners (including saccharin, aspartame [NutraSweet], and cyclamates). Almost every one of these additives has been shown to have a potential health risk.

Perhaps our biggest problem with food is our enormous American appetite. We eat about 40 percent more calories than we need, and obesity (weighing 20 percent above ideal body weight) has become epidemic. A massive nine-year U.S. study on caloric intake involving two dozen laboratories, sixty government and university researchers, and 24,000 rats and mice is currently in its fifth year. The results of restricting caloric intake by 40 percent have had a dramatic impact on increasing longevity. The most prominent advocate of human caloric restriction is Roy L. Wolford, M.D., an immunologist at the University of California at Los Angeles, who has raised some of the world's oldest mice using caloric restriction. His findings are described in his books *Maximum Lifespan* and *The 120-Year Diet*.

Our society has chosen food as its greatest treat, and unfortunately, the most highly prized foods not only have no nutritional value but ultimately can make us sick. Now that I have eliminated many of your life's greatest pleasures—ice cream, soda pop, sugar, coffee, and alcohol—as well as 40 percent of your calories, I hope you are still with me. I'm sorry. I can tell you, though, that when I stopped eating ice cream nearly five years ago, I thought it would be a lot more difficult than it turned out to be. What happens is that shortly after making these dietary changes, you will begin to appreciate new rewards: more energy, less mucus, fewer pounds, and a great feeling of accomplishment that comes from applying self-discipline toward doing something beneficial for yourself. Remember, too, that these are just recommendations, not commandments. My own guideline on this subject is "Everything in moderation, including moderation." I do believe, however, that if you are miserable with sick sinuses you should try to adhere as closely as possible to these suggestions. Try to make at least a three-month commitment to this diet.

A healthy diet is generally rich in fruits, fresh vegetables, whole grains (e.g., brown rice, bulgur wheat or kashi, oats, millet, quinoa, lupina, and whole-wheat noodles), legumes, and fiber (abundant in bran cereals, beans, apricots, and prunes). Raw foods are usually better than cooked. Good sources of protein are nuts, seeds, fish, turkey, chicken, and the soybean products tofu and tempeh. The foods that most strengthen the immune system are also highly beneficial to those whose sinus condition is caused by nasal allergies; these are garlic, onions, citrus fruits, and horseradish.

This is only a brief discussion of nutrition. Classes on the subject or consultation with a nutritionist would help you tailor a healthy diet to your personal tastes. Two books often recommended by nutritionists are *Food Is Your Best Medicine* by Henry G. Bieler, M.D., and *Vibrant Health from Your Kitchen* by Bernard Jensen.

If you have followed the preceding recommendations without a noticeable improvement in your condition, I suggest eliminating from your diet for at least three weeks the foods that most commonly produce the allergic reactions that might cause chronic sinusitis: cow's milk and all dairy products, wheat, chocolate, corn, white sugar, soy, yeast (brewer's and baker's), oranges, tomatoes, bell peppers, white potatoes, eggs, garlic, peanuts, black pepper, red meat, coffee, black tea, beer, wine, and champagne. I realize how difficult this can be, but it only need be for three weeks. After that, begin to reintroduce each of these foods into your diet at the rate of one every three days. Pay attention to your body and note any new symptoms such as headache, nausea, diarrhea, gas, or mental "fog." It then should be obvious to you which food, if any, causes your body to react. If you suspect food sensitivities, or suffer from hypoglycemia or chronic fatigue, the book *High Energy* by Rob Krakovitz, M.D., is an excellent resource.

I wish there were some way to make dietary change both simple and easy. If there were, I am sure it wouldn't have taken so many years for my family's diet to have reached the healthy point it has—and even that was with the added impetus of my daughter Carin's wish to be a vegetarian. If there is a good health-food store not too far from your home, try to shop there. The salespeople are usually very helpful. Many supermarkets now have health-food sections. Take a few extra minutes on your next trip to see what looks good. Be a little adventuresome, but do try to implement change gradually. This transition should not be made in two weeks. Those who take their time have a much greater chance of maintaining their healthy diet. Although there are many powerful therapeutic measures to help your sinuses, few are more valuable than eating only food that is nourishing to your body.

WATER

Water has been called our most essential nutrient. Regular water drinking might be the simplest, least expensive self-help measure for the maintenance of good health.

The percentage of water in a human body varies from 60 to 80 percent. At birth, a baby's body is about 80 percent water, and the average adult's body is between 60 and 70 percent. Every bodily function occurs through the medium of water. Water helps to cleanse the blood by removing wastes through the kidneys; it is vital to digestion and metabolism; it is crucial to nerve impulse conduction; it carries nutrients and oxygen to the cells through the blood; it helps to regulate our body temperature through perspiration; it lubricates our joints; and as I have already mentioned, the respiratory tract needs it to lubricate the mucous membrane. The sinuses drain more easily when you are well hydrated and their mucous membrane is more resistant to infection.

Unfortunately, many Americans are chronically dehydrated. This condition can impair every aspect of the body's normal functioning, resulting in reduced blood volume with less oxygen and nutrients provided to all muscles and organs, excess body fat, poor muscle tone and size, decreased digestive efficiency (constipation), increased toxicity in the body, joint and muscle soreness (especially after exercise), and water retention (the body retains water to compensate for the shortage). This is why proper water intake is important for weight loss. In general, we need to drink more water than our thirst calls for.

A healthy but sedentary adult weighing 160 pounds should drink about ten 8-ounce glasses of water a day (one-half ounce per pound of body weight); an active, athletic person of the same weight should drink thirteen to fourteen 8-ounce glasses a day (two-thirds ounce per pound). Try to spread your intake throughout the day (it's best to drink between meals), and don't drink more than four glasses in any given hour. Don't substitute beer, coffee, tea, soft drinks, or processed fruit juice for pure water. Although they all contain water, they also have other ingredients that can negate the positive effect of water. Herbal tea, natural fruit juices (without sugar and diluted 50 percent with water), and some soups (low salt, no sugar, the clearer and thinner the better) can substitute for a portion of your daily water requirement. Often overlooked is the fact that we also obtain water by absorbing it through our skin while bathing and showering.

Water quality is so variable in the United States that it is impossible to generalize about whether you should drink tap, bottled, or filtered water. I don't recommend distilled water for drinking because it doesn't provide the necessary minerals. In some communities the water is so pure they don't even need to treat it; other sources contain high levels of lead and radon, the two worst contaminants. Radon can cause cancer, and lead can impair the development of brain cells in children. Unfortunately, you can't depend on the local government to protect you from water pollution. According to Gene Rosov, president of WaterTest Corporation, the nation's largest independent drinking-water testing laboratory, "The majority of the health-related risks that are present in drinking water are a result of the contamination added *after* the water leaves the treatment and distribution plant." This means that it would be a good idea to have the water at your tap tested, regardless of your local water utility's claims about water quality. Call your health department for a referral for testing. Reverse-osmosis filters appear to be the most effective home water-filtering systems presently available.

It is a fact of life in America today that we can never know for certain whether what we drink or eat is completely safe. Do the best you can. Remember to drink more water and to make it convenient (keep a water container in your car and at your desk while working). Don't wait until you're thirsty to drink, and most important, be sure that there's always a bathroom nearby.

VITAMINS, HERBS, AND NUTRITIONAL SUPPLEMENTS

In case you hadn't noticed, life in urban America can be extremely stressful. Almost daily we are exposed to chemical stress, emotional stress, and infection. Each type of stress has numerous sources. Chemical stress, for example, may come from polluted air, polluted water, food pesticides, insecticides, heavy metals, or, worst of all, radioactive wastes. All stresses harm us by weakening our immune systems with highly toxic molecules called free radicals. According to Deepak Chopra, M.D., author of *Quantum Healing: Exploring the Frontiers of Mind/Body Medicine*, free radicals are the "metabolic end-products in the body of environmental pollution, food toxins, carcinogens, and emotional toxins."

Medical research has already implicated free radicals as causative factors in many diseases (e.g., arthritis, mental disorders, and heart disease), as well as in susceptibility to infection and in the process of aging. In fact, over the past thirty years, research has revealed a common factor in every degenerative disease of our time: cell damage as a result of free radicals. Denham Harman, M.D., of the University of Nebraska says, "Today it seems very likely that the assumption that there is a basic cause of aging is correct and that the sum of deleterious free radical reactions going on continuously throughout the cells and tissues is the aging process or a major contribution to it."

Free radicals are responsible for most cellular damage. Fortunately, our bodies manufacture antioxidant enzymes within the cells for protection against free radicals, and also employ antioxidant nutrients (e.g., vitamin A [beta-carotene], vitamin E, and vitamin C) supplied by our diet. As long as there is an adequate supply of oxygen, water, antioxidant nutrients, and enzymes in the body, cell damage is minimized. When any one of these is deficient, cell damage is accelerated, as in the process of aging and in disease. Through their critical role in helping to prevent disease, vitamins, acting as antioxidants, can offer considerable help to our body's immune system.

When disease, including chronic sinusitis, is present, the cells are overrun with an excess of free radicals and the immune system cannot maintain its protective shield. This occurs when stress lowers our body's production of antioxidant enzymes to a level less than our needs. Unfortunately, city living makes it difficult to avoid most of our stressors. It is a wonder that the majority of us are free of a chronic disease. For those who have not been as fortunate, and for anyone interested in strengthening their body's natural defenses, practicing preventive medicine, or experiencing a greater degree of physical health, the following recommendations for vitamins, herbs, and nutritional supplements will help.

Vitamin C

In 1970 the distinguished chemist and Nobel Prize winner Linus Pauling turned his attention to the benefits of megadoses of vitamin C in the prevention and treatment of colds. The verification of his findings by other researchers has been complicated primarily by the great variability in the dosages and types of vitamin C that have been used. In my experience, vitamin C has been extremely effective in the treatment and prevention of both colds and sinus infections. In that colds are the most common cause of acute sinusitis, their prevention is good preventive medicine for sinusitis. In addition to its antioxidant properties, vitamin C is essential to the manufacture of collagen, the main supportive protein of skin, tendon, bone, cartilage, and connective tissue; has an anti-inflammatory effect, especially in some autoimmune diseases such as lupus and rheumatoid arthritis; facilitates the absorption of dietary iron; enhances the immune response and white blood cell activity; and, in conjunction with vitamin E, strengthens arterial walls and provides greater protection against cholesterol buildup and heart disease.

The average daily dose for cold prevention is 3,000 milligrams (mg). If you already have a cold or sinus infection, I recommend as much as 15,000 mg a day. Take this amount in divided dosages, either 5,000 mg three times a day with meals (to avoid stomach upset, it is best to take most vitamins with food) or 2,000 to 3,000 mg every two to three hours, preferably in a powdered form as ascorbate. This is much more easily absorbed and more potent than ascorbic acid—the more common form of vitamin C found in fruits, vegetables, and most commercial brands of vitamin C. You can also take time-released vitamin C capsules or tablets that are assimilated over twelve hours. Most other vitamin C tablets last for only six to eight hours. This high dosage for colds and sinus infections should be maintained for about one week, or until your symptoms begin to improve. Taper off very gradually over the next two weeks to get back down to the usual daily dose of 3,000 mg. Possible side effects of dosages above 3,000 mg are diarrhea, bowel gas, and cramps. But these symptoms are more likely to occur with the pure ascorbic acid form of vitamin C. If you experience these symptoms, cut back on your next dose by 1,000 mg. A less common side effect is the development of kidney stones. This can usually be prevented by drinking the recommended daily amount of water or by taking 75 mg of vitamin B_6 a day.

Another method for taking vitamin C, called titrating to bowel tolerance, was developed by Robert Cathcart, M.D. Cathcart has treated over 9,000 patients with large doses of ascorbic acid, some as great as 100,000 mg a day. He believes the maximum relief of symptoms is obtained at a point just short of the amount that produces diarrhea. According to Dr. Cathcart, the amount of vitamin C that can be taken orally without causing diarrhea when a person is ill might be as much as ten times the amount he or she would tolerate if well. Using this method, he claims success treating a host of viral infections, including colds, influenza, mononucleosis, and viral pneumonia; environmental and food allergies; cancer; rheumatoid arthritis; hepatitis; and yeast infections.

There is quite a variation in the strength of different brands of vitamin C. For instance, 1,000 mg of ascorbate is better absorbed than 1,000 mg of ascorbic acid. Once ascorbic acid is absorbed into our bloodstream, it reacts with many minerals, such as sodium, calcium, magnesium, and zinc, to form ascorbates. It is in this form, as ascorbates, that vitamin C enters the trillions of cells in our bodies. The commercial brands of C that I recommend are Natrol (Ester C); Alacer Super Gram II timed release or the powder Emergen-C; Ethical Nutrients esterified polyascorbate; and Nature's Plus Ascorbate C. Taking vitamin C in ascorbate powder is the most effective way to enhance absorption.

Vitamin C, as an antioxidant, is a free-radical scavenger. Our bodies can use a lot more of it when we are under stress. Use your own discretion in varying your dosage, depending on the degree of stress you think you have experienced that day. If it was a high air pollution day or if you had a rough time at work, take more than the 3,000 mg. The same recommendation holds true for all of the other vitamins and herbs I will mention in the following sections. Vitamin C and all of the other vitamins and herbs are more effective if eaten in the natural form of food rather than taken in pill or powder forms. The foods highest in vitamin C are red chili peppers, red sweet peppers, green sweet peppers, kale, parsley, collard greens, turnip greens, mustard greens, broccoli, brussels sprouts, cauliflower, guavas, oranges, cantaloupe, and strawberries. Their vitamin C content is higher when eaten raw.

Vitamin A and Beta-Carotene

Most vitamin A comes from its precursor, beta-carotene, which is converted to the vitamin form in the gastrointestinal tract. Beta-carotene is a substance in carotenoids, which are usually found in yellow, orange, or red foods. Listed in roughly descending order of vitamin A content, these include carrots, sweet potatoes, yams, kale, spinach, mangoes, winter squash, cantaloupe, apricots, broccoli, romaine lettuce, asparagus, tomatoes, nectarines, peaches, and papayas. Vitamin A itself can be obtained directly from consumption of cod liver oil, liver, kidney, eggs, and dairy products.

Vitamin A helps to maintain the integrity of mucous membranes, is required for growth and repair of cells, is necessary for protein metabolism, protects night vision, and protects against cancer. Beta-carotene has been shown to have an effect as an anticancer nutrient—a discovery made by Japanese researchers more than twenty years ago. It is also a powerful antioxidant and a potent immunostimulator. In recent research conducted by Charles Hennekens, M.D., of Harvard Medical School, beta-carotene was found to reduce dramatically (by 50 percent) strokes and heart attacks in people who already have cardiovascular disease. Adequate beta-carotene in the diet should supply the vitamin A you need, but vitamin A deficiency in the United States is not uncommon. According to a survey by the U.S. Department of Health, Education, and Welfare, about 60 percent of women and 50 percent of men have intakes below the standard set for good nutrition. Pure vitamin A can be toxic to the liver in prolonged dosages greater than 50,000 I.U. (international units) a day, but beta-carotene is not. The only side effect of high doses of beta-carotene is yellowing skin, which is not dangerous and disappears when levels are reduced. For sinus infections it is recommended that you take beta-carotene at 50,000 I.U. two times a day. After the infection (acute or chronic) has been resolved, this dosage can be cut in half and continued indefinitely.

Vitamin E

The specific functions of vitamin E are unclear. It has recently been recognized as an antioxidant and in some studies has been shown to raise levels of the desirable cholesterol, HDL. According to Nabil Elsayed, Ph.D., a professor of public health at UCLA, "You will definitely improve your chances of resisting smog if you increase your vitamin E intake." He believes that vitamin E can significantly reduce lung damage from ozone. For people with sinusitis, 400 I.U. of vitamin E daily are recommended. When it is combined with selenium, vitamin E becomes twice as potent. This dosage need not be reduced as the symptoms of the infection subside. Foods highest in vitamin E are crude and unrefined soybean oil and wheat germ oil, fresh wheat germ, whole grains, raw nuts (most varieties), and all green, leafy vegetables.

Multivitamins

There are many comparable multivitamins from which to choose. Make sure your choice has all of the B vitamins. Take one daily whether you have sinusitis or not, and in addition to the vitamin supplements A, C, and E.

Minerals

The two minerals that seem most effective in aiding the body's immune system are selenium and zinc. A recent article in the *Journal of the National Cancer Institute* said that men with lower levels of selenium in their blood were most likely to develop cancers of the lung, stomach, and pancreas. Low selenium levels might also be linked to bladder cancer and asthma. To treat symptomatic sinus infections I recommend either selenium citrate, aspartate, or picolinate in a dosage of 195 micrograms (mcg) daily; or selenium in a combination pill with vitamin E. Foods high in selenium are whole-wheat products, fish, whole grains, mushrooms, beans, garlic, and liver. Selenium can be toxic to the body, so don't maintain a daily dosage greater than 200 mcg for longer than two weeks. Then reduce it to a maintenance dosage between 100 to 150.

Zinc appears to be critical to the release of vitamin A from the liver and is vital to the process by which new cells are produced and protein metabolized for repair of body tissues.

People with sinusitis should take 15 mg of zinc picolinate or oratate three times a day, but only when symptomatic. The foods highest in zinc are beef liver and the dark meat of turkey. The recommended maintenance dosage of zinc is 15 mg, which can be taken in your multivitamin.

Herbs, Botanicals, and Other Remedies

It has been estimated that nearly 25 percent of all pharmaceutical drugs are made from plants, herbs, leaves, bark, or roots. In September 1990, cancer researchers asked the Department of the Interior for federal protection for the Pacific yew, a tree found in the ancient forests of the Pacific Northwest whose bark provides a scarce new cancer-fighting drug. The fact that we are destroying global forests so rapidly, especially the rain forests, means that we are eliminating potentially life-saving drugs without even knowing it. Many species of plants are becoming extinct before botanists can determine their value. There are still a few human cultures remaining that depend almost entirely on naturally occurring vegetation for their medicines.

Onions; the herbs garlic, echinacea, and goldenseal; and bee propolis all seem to strengthen the immune system to such an extent that they might be called natural antibiotics. I recommend all of them to patients with both acute and chronic sinusitis (types 1 and 2). They can be taken in addition to a pharmaceutical antibiotic in the form of a capsule, liquid, or tea. Good reference books for medicinal herbs are *A Textbook of Natural Medicine* by Joseph Pizzorno, N.D., and *The Complete Botanical Prescriber* by John Sherman, N.D.

Garlic, a member of the lily family, is a perennial plant, cultivated around the world, that has been prescribed throughout history to treat a variety of ailments. Egyptians have been using it for almost 5,000 years, and the Chinese for at least 3,000 years. Hippocrates and Aristotle cited many therapeutic uses for garlic, including the relief of coughs, toothache, earache, dandruff, hypertension, atherosclerosis, diarrhea and dysentery, and vaginitis. It can be effective as an antibacterial, antiviral, antifungal, antihypertensive, and anti-inflammatory agent. At the National Cancer Institute garlic has recently shown promise in fighting stomach and colon cancer. Garlic is for the most part nontoxic, although it does cause bad breath. Many brands of processed garlic are available at health-food stores in pill, capsule, and liquid forms. Raw garlic is best, up to one clove per day.

Echinacea is at the top of the list of immunity-enhancing herbs. A perennial herb native to the American Midwest, it serves as an immunostimulator, wound healer and anti-inflammatory, antiviral, antibacterial, and antineoplastic (cancer). It can be taken alone or in a liquid combination with goldenseal, in a dosage of forty drops three times a day. It also comes in capsules. Think of echinacea as you would an anti-biotic. It must be taken regularly in order to have a therapeutic effect, but if taken beyond three months you can build up a tolerance to its therapeutic effect.

Goldenseal is a perennial herb native to eastern North America and is cultivated in Oregon and Washington state. It is best known for its action in soothing inflammatory conditions of the respiratory, digestive, and genitourinary tracts caused by allergy or infection. It enhances the function of the mucous membranes. Goldenseal should not be taken by women who are pregnant or who plan a pregnancy in the near future. People with known or suspected hypoglycemia and certain weed pollen allergies should also avoid taking it without medical supervision. There is also considered to be a minimal risk to children and people over age fifty-five with the use of goldenseal, and it should not be taken in large quantities for extended periods of time. With acute sinusitis, you can take twenty to thirty drops three times a day.

Bee propolis is an extract from the bee's body (it is *not*

bee pollen), and it comes in both liquid and capsules. The dosage is 500 mg three times a day. If you use the liquid form, follow the instructions on the bottle. Bee propolis appears to enhance immune function.

There are a growing number of products available containing the herb ephedra, a natural decongestant, from which many of the pharmaceutical decongestants have been derived. The following products (with the name of the company in parentheses) contain ephedra in combination with other beneficial herbs: Sinustop (Nature's Way), HAS (Nature's Way), and Sinus-Ade (Dr. Clayton). There are others. One that does not contain ephedra but has many other medicinal herbs helpful for both sinusitis and allergies is Cobiozin (Great Life Lab). After selecting one of these, you should follow the dosage instructions on the package. Those on heart or blood pressure medications should only take these under medical supervision.

Recently, several vitamin companies have introduced products that combine many of the antioxidants with other medicinal herbs. If any are available at your health-food store, you might be able to fulfill the foregoing recommendations with just one type of tablet or capsule.

For readers whose primary complaint is a terrible postnasal drip, or just a lot of clear nasal mucus drainage without a sinus infection, I recently learned of an effective remedy: fish oil. It can be found in the store as Super EPA (300 mg). Begin with a dosage of two or three capsules a day, then add one a day up to eight or ten capsules or until your symptoms have improved. Then maintain this dosage for at least a month before gradually tapering back down to one capsule a day. If you are a good candidate for the fish oil treatment, you might have several of the following symptoms: dry eyes; dry mouth or excessive thirst; becoming easily cold or easily overheated; dry skin everywhere except face and scalp, which are too oily; cracking on the sides of your heels and fingertips; breaking of fingernails (in layers); rough skin on your thighs, buttocks, and the backs of your arms. The most common side effect of this treatment is belching. This can be minimized by refrigerating the capsules and taking them cold. Diarrhea and a flulike syndrome are also possibilities. Fish oil has also been found to be effective for the treatment of arthritis and chronic urticaria (hives).

Two other natural remedies for chronic sinusitis are peppermint oil and camphorated salve (Tiger Balm). I put a very small amount (one drop) of peppermint oil on my fingertip, then wipe it around the *outside* of both nostrils. The oil, which acts as a stimulant, seems to improve circulation to the nasal and sinus mucous membranes. This enhances the effect of breathing clean and moist air. I like to spray my nose with the saline spray or stand in front of the humidifier and then apply the peppermint oil. It feels wonderful! Eucalyptus oil has a similar effect. The Tiger Balm seems to work on the same principle for your lungs. With a sinus infection I recommend applying it to your chest two or three times a day.

ALLERGY TREATMENT

In Chapter 5 I discussed the traditional medical approach to the treatment of allergies or allergic rhinitis. If you are interested in a complement to that regimen or in a non-medicated alternative, it is possible to treat allergies effectively without drugs. I would recommend a very similar holistic program to the one for sinus disease. An air cleaner or negative ion generator to remove airborne allergens is an important first step. The diet is the same as for sinus sufferers with an emphasis on those fruits and vegetables with the highest content of antioxidants. Modified cleansing diets are also helpful during your high allergy season. These should be administered by a nutritionally oriented physician or a naturopath. Ruling out food allergy is another suggestion. Many people with pollen allergy are also allergic to foods, particularly dairy and wheat.

The dosages for the vitamin supplements are also the same as for sinusitis, but instead of taking the higher amounts for a sinus infection you would take them preventively during the allergy season or whenever you experience a flare-up of your allergy symptoms. In addition to vitamin C (in an ascorbate form), vitamin E plus selenium, beta-carotene, and a multivitamin; for allergies I also suggest acidophilus (same dosage as for yeast treatment), vitamin B_6 200 mg twice per day, and pantothenic acid 500 mg three times per day following meals. A natural antihistamine called Antronex can be taken twice per day. If your health-food store doesn't have it, they may be able to order it from the manufacturer, Standard Process, or you can also ask your local chiropractor to obtain it for you.

Perhaps the most exciting development in nutritional science for the treatment of allergies is the bioflavinoid quercetin. Blue-green algae are the usual source of this substance, but it is also available as a food supplement. Quercetin is safe, nontoxic, and barely soluble in water, so poor dietary absorption may limit its efficacy. Because of this it is suggested that it be taken in combination with bromelain to improve its absorption. Bromelain is a natural, protein-digesting enzyme derived from pineapples. It has been used to increase absorption of a wide variety of compounds, including antibiotics.

The total daily dosage of quercetin should be between 1,000 and 2,000 mg divided into three to six doses. In addition to the treatment of allergies, quercetin has also been used with some success for asthma.

In the chapters that follow you will learn the mental, emotional, spiritual, and social aspects of the holistic program for the treatment of chronic sinusitis as well as allergies and any other chronic ailment. Please make a note of the specific affirmation used for allergies and the reflexology points found on the hands and feet specifically for the nose. The acupressure points on the face for the treatment of sinusitis can also be used for allergies.

EXERCISE

No discussion of physical health would be complete without including the subject of exercise. Americans live in a relatively sedentary society. We watch an average of more than four hours of television every day, and only 36 percent of our children are required to take physical education classes in school. The majority of adults cite lack of time as the most common reason for not exercising. Studies have shown that sedentary people, on average, don't live as long or enjoy as good health as those who get regular aerobic exercise: brisk walking, running, swimming, cycling, or similar workouts. Some researchers now believe that getting no exercise might be a more significant risk factor for decreased life expectancy than the *combined* risk of cigarette smoking, high cholesterol, overweight, and high blood pressure.

The word *aerobic* literally means "with oxygen," and is used to refer to prolonged exercise that requires extra oxygen to supply energy to the muscles through the metabolizing of carbohydrates and fat. This is the type of exercise that produces the greatest benefits to the cardiovascular system as well as to every other part of the body. The long-term results include slower heart rate, greater cardiac (heart) efficiency, lower blood pressure, and greater physical fitness. Following an aerobic workout, more oxygen is able to reach every cell in every organ of the body. If you are looking to decrease the effects of chronic sinusitis (or any other chronic condition) and attain a greater overall feeling of well-being, I recommend a regular program of aerobic exercise.

This does *not* have to entail a great deal of time. Keep in mind the factors of fun ("What activity would I like to do?" or "What might feel good to me?") and convenience ("How can this be done in the least amount of time?" or "How can I best fit this into my schedule?"). A minimum program of aerobic exercise need consist of only three thirty-minute workouts weekly, maintaining your fitness heart rate two-thirds of that time. To determine this heart rate, use the following formula: 220 minus your age multiplied by 65 to 85 percent equals your fitness heart rate. For example, a 40-year-old's fitness heart rate is between 117 and 153 beats per minute. You have to know how to take your pulse (using your index and middle fingers, feel the pulse either on the thumb side of your wrist or at your neck just below the jaw) and you need a watch with a second hand. Count the number of beats in six seconds and multiply that number by ten to determine your heart rate in beats per minute. When you have attained your fitness heart rate (after about five to ten minutes of exercising), try to maintain it for at least twenty minutes. It is also beneficial to cool down (slower heart rate and less intensity of exercise) for five to ten minutes following the twenty minutes at the fitness rate.

The most convenient forms of aerobic exercise involving the least amount of wear and tear on the body are brisk walking, hiking, swimming, and cycling. If you have easy access to regular cross-country skiing, add that to the list. I no longer recommend running, after seeing too many patients with running-related complaints, usually involving the knees and feet. For year-round cycling, try either a good ten-speed with a turbo trainer for indoor cycling or a stationary bike. Treadmill, rowing, stair-climb, and cross-country ski machines also offer an opportunity for excellent indoor aerobic exercise, as do low-impact aerobics classes. There are several sports played one-on-one or in teams—such as racquetball, handball, badminton, tennis (singles), and basketball—that have the po-

tential for providing a good aerobic workout. Exercise outdoors if you live or work where it is convenient and safe to do
so (specifically with regard to automobile traffic and outdoor
air quality and temperature). The combination of fresh air
and sunshine provides greater benefits than indoor exercise.
For chronic sinus sufferers, and for those practicing sinus disease prevention, air quality is a critical factor in determining
where and when to exercise. Ozone, the most harmful of air
pollutants, is created by the combination of nitrogen oxides,
hydrocarbons, and sunlight. A bright sunny day in the down-
town area of most large cities would produce high concentrations of ozone. The EPA considers air unhealthy when ozone
levels top 0.125 parts per million. However, in a study conducted by New York University's Morton Lippman, M.D.,
thirty healthy adults showed decreases in lung capacity during
a half-hour of exercise at ozone levels below the federal limit.

Writing in the May/June 1989 issue of the journal *Hippocrates*, Benedict Carey suggested scheduling exercise around
the rise and fall of pollution levels. In the summer, Carey
noted, ozone builds up during the morning, reaches its maximum late in the afternoon, and then ebbs in the evening. In
the winter, ozone isn't such a problem, but cold night air can
trap a layer of carbon monoxide, nitrogen dioxide, sulfur dioxide, and particulates that can linger into the early morning. A
good general practice is to do outdoor exercise in the morning
during the summer and in the evening during the winter.

If you are used to walking, biking, or jogging along main
roads, lung specialists recommend that you stay away from
these high-traffic areas during rush hour. Avoid waiting beside
stop signs or stoplights, where carbon monoxide builds up.
Henry Going, M.D., a UCLA pulmonologist, says, "I've seen
guys jogging in place next to cars at stoplights. You might as
well smoke a cigarette." On windy days pollution disperses
quickly as you move away from the road. On calm days it can

extend about sixty feet from either side of the road.

If all of these concerns pose too great an obstacle, if you live in a highly polluted city, or if you experience a wheeze, cough, or tightness in your chest during your workout, it's time to head indoors for aerobic exercise. Ozone levels in most homes, gyms, and pools are about half that of the outdoors— even less with a good air-conditioning system.

William S. Silvers, M.D., a Denver allergist, has found that many patients with respiratory difficulties who exercise regularly and follow this with a wet steam exposure experience improved breathing, increased mucus flow and expectoration, and had less nasal and throat congestion. He recommends that following your twenty to thirty minutes of aerobic exercise, and after your heart rate has dropped to its pre-exercise level, you have five to ten minutes of exposure to wet steam. This can be done in either a steam room at a health club, the bathroom of your home, or by standing over a boiling pot of water with a towel over your head. You should do nasal/chest breathing, which is best performed by taking a deep, slow inhalation through your nose and then breathing out from your chest. Do this as many days as you can, whether you exercise indoors or outdoors.

Moderate exercise is less strenuous than aerobic but still beneficial. In a recent research project at the University of Minnesota School of Public Health, moderate exercise was defined as rapid walking, bowling, gardening, yard work, home repairs, dancing, and home exercise, conducted for about an hour daily. A treadmill test determined that those who got this much leisure-time exercise had healthier hearts than those who got less or none. There was no added benefit in doing more than an hour's worth of physical activity. Robert E. Thayer, Ph.D., a professor of psychology at California State University, Long Beach, has found that brisk walks only ten minutes long can increase people's feelings of energy (sometimes for several hours), reduce tension, and make personal problems appear less serious.

For strengthening and toning, I recommend both push-ups and sit-ups. Remember that with sit-ups you need not raise your trunk any higher than 45 degrees from the floor.

Maintaining and increasing flexibility is an essential part of your overall physical fitness program. Flexibility is the ability to use muscles and joints through their full range of movement. Research has suggested that good muscle elasticity lends agility, a potential for greater speed, and a reduced chance of injury to muscles, tendons, and ligaments. A regular routine of gentle stretching or yoga can be a relaxing and invigorating way to start your day. The books *Stretching* by Bob Anderson, and *Yoga: The Iyengar Way* by Mira, Silva, and Shyam Mehta, are both excellent guides.

Aerobic exercise was an integral part of the program I used to cure my own chronic sinusitis, and it is still a big part of my routine. Initially it requires discipline. Start gradually and try not to push yourself too hard. Exercise does not have to hurt to be beneficial, in spite of the prevalent belief in "no pain, no gain." It won't take long before you start looking forward to it as one of the highlights of your day. The benefits that you will soon realize will help to increase your motivation to continue. You might eventually make it a daily routine, although research has shown no increased cardiovascular benefits beyond five days a week (three times a week is minimum). However, exercise does much more than merely benefit your heart. As these aerobic workouts strengthen your heart and lungs directly, your ability to provide oxygen to every part of your body is enhanced—and this, after all, is the scientific basis of physical health. As a human animal, you can experience many of life's greatest pleasures only through your body. Regular exercise can add immeasurably to your enjoyment of life and heighten your sense of well-being.

PHYSICAL HEALTH RECOMMENDATIONS: A SUMMARY

Those recommendations marked with an asterisk are to be taken only for sinus infections or other acute conditions.

- Follow the treatment program recommended by your physician. This might include antibiotics, decongestants, moisture and irrigation, and any of the other elements of the treatment for acute sinusitis mentioned in Chapter 4.
- Make an attempt to breathe air that is clean, moist, warm, and rich in oxygen and negative ions.
- Maintain a diet that is rich in fresh vegetables, fruit, whole grains, legumes and fiber. Avoid dairy products, sugar, caffeine, and red meat.
- Drink about eight to ten 8-ounce glasses of clean water (or one-half ounce per pound of body weight) on days you are not exercising. Drink fourteen to sixteen 8-ounce glasses (or two-thirds ounce per pound of body weight) on days you are exercising.
- Take vitamin C at 5,000 mg three times a day for about one week or until there is a noticeable improvement in your sinus infection, and then gradually taper off this amount over the next two weeks to 1,000 mg three times a day as a maintenance dose.
- Take beta-carotene, 50,000 I.U. two times a day until the infection clears, and then 25,000 I.U. two times a day for maintenance.
- Take vitamin E, 400 I.U. daily, or preferably in combination with selenium.
- Take a multivitamin, one daily.
- Take garlic,* 2 capsules three times a day.
- Take echinacea with goldenseal,* 40 drops three times a day.

- Take selenium citrate or selenium aspartate,* 195
  mcg daily (or 100 to 150 mcq daily in combination
  with vitamin E).
- Take zinc picolinate,* 15 mg three times a day.
- Take bee propolis,* 500 mg three times a day.
- Use peppermint oil and Tiger Balm; apply two times
  a day.
- Engage in aerobic exercise for 30 minutes (at least 20
  minutes at your fitness heart rate) three to five times
  a week. Your fitness heart rate = (220 − your age)
  × 65 to 85 percent. Exercise can be brisk walking,
  swimming, cycling, or indoor machines: treadmill,
  rowing, stair-climb, or cross-country ski.

With the exception of the prescription drugs and most of the
herbs and minerals, this is a program that can be continued
indefinitely, long after your sinus condition has gone. The vitamins I still take on a daily basis are 3,000 mg of vitamin C,
beta-carotene at 50,000 I.U., vitamin E at 200 I.U. plus selenium at 120 mcg, and a multivitamin. I have learned, just as
you will, to become much more sensitive to my body. Whenever I feel weak or am exposed to environmental or stressful
conditions that are unhealthy to my sinuses, I take more of the
vitamins and herbs (or eat more food with these nutrients in
them) and increase my dosage of vitamin C.

This approach combines elements of the "quick fix" with
preventive medicine. I realize that many of the recommendations entail making changes in your daily habits. However,
if you are willing to make the commitment and purchase the
machines to improve indoor air, modify your diet, drink more
water, exercise more often, and take the prescribed list of vitamins and herbs, I guarantee that your chronic sinusitis will
improve. I have seen many patients who were able to stop taking long-term antibiotics, decongestants, antihistamines, cortisone, decongestant and cortisone nasal sprays, and asthma

medications after adhering to this regimen for several months. In that many of these people had been on their medications for several years, I considered this a quick fix. The patients considered it something close to a miracle. However, there is nothing miraculous about it. Physical health is quite basic.

11 MENTAL HEALTH

The breadth of the term *mental health* is so great it almost defies definition. In my opinion, true mental health means that you are both aware of and are practicing your gifts and special talents; recognizing the extent to which your thoughts, beliefs, attitudes, and mental pictures limit or expand your potential to enjoy life; learning to make choices based on your intuition; attaining some degree of clarity regarding your priorities, values, and goals; working at a job that you enjoy; and incorporating humor, forgiveness, gratitude, and hope into your life. The end result is a condition that combines peace of mind with living your dreams.

It is not within the scope of this book to explore any of these areas in great depth. I would, however, like you to become more aware of how your mental health affects your physical health, and to learn some simple things that will help you attain a greater degree of mental fitness.

BELIEFS, AFFIRMATIONS, GOALS, AND NLP

Most patients who come to see me have already sought help from one or even several physicians. Their doctors have told them, "You're going to have to live with your sinus problem"; "You have six months left to live with that cancer"; "Your back/sinus/knee requires surgery"; or "There's nothing more that can be done for it" (the majority of diseases). These statements are, however, only beliefs. The beliefs are based on the limitations of modern medical science, a highly scientific and technologically advanced approach to the treatment of disease, and they are delivered to the patient by a highly educated individual in a society that defers to expertise. These pronouncements, which are in some cases death sentences, are quickly accepted by most patients and become a part of their own belief system. The vast majority of people with terminal diseases who accept whatever their doctors tell them (these patients are called "compliant") die very close to the predicted time. Patients who challenge prognoses tend to live longer. In *Love, Medicine and Miracles,* Bernie Siegel, M.D., vividly describes how the beliefs and attitudes of many of his cancer patients affected the outcome of their disease.

Most of the beliefs held by Americans have been defined by the standards, or norms, of our society, but how well does the norm fit you, a unique individual? If all of us attempted to conform, the world would be a boring place, devoid of creativity and innovation. We certainly wouldn't be enjoying the ease of living that technology has provided us were it not for the adventuresome few who deviated from the conventional belief system.

Unfortunately, in every culture there is great pressure to conform. It isn't easy, to say the least, to hold beliefs that run counter to prevalent attitudes. Society, friends, and family all tell us we have strayed with phrases such as "you should," "you ought to," or—if your belief has caused them a lot of discomfort—"you're crazy!" Most of the time we respond to this pressure by giving up our unreasonable, or even outrageous, belief. Ultimately, all of us would prefer to be accepted and loved by others; besides, we tell ourselves, "it wasn't that big a deal anyway."

Your belief system has a profound impact on your life: what you eat and think, how you dress and behave, what you do for a living, how you spend your leisure time, what your values and goals are, and how you define health and quality of life. It also determines the nature of the silent messages you give yourself every day. All of us talk to ourselves, and this internal dialogue has a great deal to do with our state of mental health. These messages might be generally self-critical ("You stupid . . ."; "Why did you say that?"; "Why did you do that?"; "How could you . . ?"; "You should've/could've . . .") ; or they might be accepting and supportive ("Good job!"; "That's fine"; "You did the best you could"). All of my patients are very hard on themselves. They are self-critical and put themselves under a great deal of unnecessary pressure.

As human beings we are imperfect; all of us make mistakes. The way we respond to these failings is what creates more, or lessens, stress in our lives. Our pattern of response is one we probably have been repeating since childhood. One way to change the pattern is through the use of verbal affirmations, positive statements that you repeat to yourself as often as possible during the day. Affirmations should be in the present tense, contain only positive words, and serve as a response to an often-heard negative message or expression of a goal.

For example, if some of the previous critical messages sound familiar to you, two affirmations that would help counteract them are: "I love and approve of myself" and "I am always doing the best I can." When people begin repeating affirmations, they usually don't believe what they're saying (that's why they're saying them), although they would like to. Using affirmations is like reprogramming a computer. Your subconscious mind is the computer that has been receiving the same message for years; now you are going to change the input.

The best time to say your affirmation is immediately following the negative message you give yourself. I remember feeling so frustrated with my sinus headaches or congestion that I would think to myself, "This will never go away." After I began affirmations, I followed my hopeless comments with an immediate "My sinuses are now completely healed." This affirmation always made me feel a little better and gave me some hope. As my condition improved, I began to believe it more and more until it was actually true. Louise Hay has written a wonderful book on self-healing called *You Can Heal Your Life*, in which she focuses on the healing potential of affirmations as a means of learning to love yourself. Ms. Hay has recently opened a clinic in Santa Monica, California, for the treatment of AIDS. Her book contains a list of medical conditions, each with a corresponding affirmation. The one for sinusitis and bronchitis is "I declare peace and harmony are within me and surround me at all times; all is well." I used that one, too, to help cure my sinus disease. For allergies she suggests, "The world is safe and friendly. I am safe. I am at peace with life." And for colds, "I allow my mind to relax and be at peace. Clarity and harmony are within me and around me."

You can use affirmations to help change any belief that doesn't feel good to you, or to help you achieve any goal. Most of my patients have come in because of one or more chronic physical or mental problems. Their objectives are clear: to stop having sinus infections, to get rid of allergies, to stop living with chronic pain, to have more energy, to suffer less anxiety, and so forth. After they have begun to see some improvement in their physical condition, I ask them to make a list of their other holistic health goals and categorize them into mental, emotional, spiritual, and social. I ask them to ask themselves: "What does the ideal future hold for me? What would it look like if I could have all of my desires met?" Their answers— more money, a job that I love, to live in a beautiful place, to experience a greater sense of freedom, to be able to better express my feelings, to have a greater intimacy in my marriage, to have a greater sense of the spiritual in my daily life—provide a blueprint for our work together. The answers also become their personal vision and give direction to their own self-healing process.

The next step is to write the answers in the form of affirmations, such as "I am living in a beautiful place," "I'm spending more time alone," or "My job is fulfilling and fun." You must be able to clarify your desires to have any chance of obtaining them and try to be as specific as possible. The next step is to believe, however minimally, that it is possible for you to meet these goals. The more you repeat the affirmations, the stronger your belief will become.

The third step in this formula for self-realization is expectation. The stronger your belief and the more objectives you have already reached, the higher will be your level of expectation. After my chronic sinusitis was resolved, I developed the belief that anything is possible, one that has helped me to realize other dreams. Whatever it is that you *desire*, as long as you *believe* it's possible, you can *expect* it to happen. It is not necessary to know how, or to have a definite plan. Just be patient and flexible and be willing to accept the result even if the package in which it arrives is different from what you had envisioned. If your objectives are clear, your intuition will help you make the right decisions to get what you want.

Schedule a time once or twice a day to recite your list of affirmations. Within a couple of weeks you will have them memorized, and you will be able to call on them anytime a negative belief or message comes up. You might want to write one or two of them on a sheet of paper on a daily basis for three weeks, or write them on a Post-it and place it in a spot that you pass by frequently. This might sound simplistic, but it is actually a powerful technique. Remember that you can always choose what to believe. Rather than continuing with the attitude, "I'll believe it when I see it," why not try, "When I believe it, then I'll see it."

How you choose to see your sinus condition or any other chronic illness can play a vital role in the way the disease affects you and whether or not it goes away. Some of the early reactions to a chronic or life-threatening disease are denial ("There must be some mistake"), anger and frustration ("Why me?"; "What terrible luck"), self-pity ("I'll never be able to enjoy life again"), and resignation ("I'll just have to put up with it and continue to live this way for the rest of my life"). All of these are quite normal and understandable responses to something as devastating as a chronic illness. However, if you are interested in healing yourself, it is important to get beyond this point and look at your disease in a different light. According to Bernie Siegel, who contributed the following material to the book *Chop Wood, Carry Water,* you have several choices:

- Accept your illness. Being resigned to an illness can be destructive and can allow the illness to run your life, but accepting it allows energy to be freed for other things in your life.
- See the illness as a source of growth. If you begin to grow psychologically in response to the loss the illness has created in your life, then you don't need to have a physical illness anymore.
- View your illness as a positive redirection in your life. This means that you don't have to judge anything that happens to you. If you get fired from a job, for example, assume that you are being redirected toward something else you are supposed to be doing. Your entire life changes when you say that something is just a redirection. You are then at peace. Everything is okay and you go on your way, knowing that the new direction is the one that is intrinsically right for you. After a while you begin to *feel* that this is true.
- Death or recurrence of illness is no longer seen as synonymous with failure after the aforementioned steps are accomplished, but simply as further choices or steps. If staying alive were your sole goal, you would have to be a failure because you do have to die someday. However, when you begin to accept the inevitability of death and see that you have only

a limited time, you begin to realize that you might as
well enjoy the present to the best of your ability.

- Learn self-love and peace of mind, and the body
responds. Your body gets "live" or "energy" messages
when you say "I love myself." That's not the ego
talking, it's self-esteem. It's as if someone else is
loving you, saying that you are a worthwhile person,
believing in you, and telling you that you are here to
give something to the world. When you do that,
your immune system says, "This person likes living;
let's fight for his or her life."

- Don't make physical change your sole goal. Seek
peace of mind, acceptance, and forgiveness. Learn to
love. In the process, the disease won't be totally
overlooked—it will be seen as one of the problems
you are having, and perhaps one of your fears. If you
learn about hope, love, acceptance, forgiveness, and
peace of mind, the disease might go away in the
process.

- Achieve immortality through love. The only way you
can live forever is to love somebody. Then you can
really leave a gift behind. When you live that way, as
many people with physical illnesses do, it is even
possible to decide when you die. You can say, "Thank
you, I've used my body to its limit. I have loved as
much as I possibly can, and I'm leaving at two
o'clock today." And you go. Then maybe you have
spent half an hour dying and the rest of your life
living; but when these things are not done, you
might spend a lot of your life dying, and only a little
living.

I realize that most of you do not have a terminal disease,
just a case of good old chronic sinusitis, but each of these options for looking at physical illness can work for you as a form
of preventive medicine. In my experience, chronic pain and
imminent death have provided the greatest motivation for

people to change, but why wait until you have reached that point of crisis?

A powerful technology for changing thoughts and beliefs is neurolinguistic programming (NLP). NLP teaches a wide variety of rapid and practical ways to change both feelings and beliefs through the use of goal setting, affirmations, and mental imagery. Developed in the early 1970s by information scientist Richard Bandler and linguistics professor John Grinder at the University of California, Santa Cruz, NLP offers a new perspective on how the mind works. It teaches us how to communicate with ourselves more powerfully by learning how to change the way we see ourselves, how we talk to ourselves, and how we feel about ourselves. It can be used as a method of therapy for eliminating unwanted responses and treating a variety of chronic ailments. It is also effective in transforming phobias and other traumatic responses; helping children and adults overcome learning disabilities; eliminating unwanted behaviors such as smoking, eating disorders, and insomnia; learning to excel in any area—sports, business, or school; and resolving conflicts between people and within yourself. NLP teaches the skills that promote positive change, which in turn can generate new possibilities and opportunities. You can learn more about NLP by reading about it in *Using Your Brain for a Change* by Richard Bandler, taking a class, or working with a certified NLP practitioner in your area.

WORK

Your job is another vital aspect of your mental health. Some questions you need to ask yourself are: "Do I enjoy my job?" "Does my work utilize my greatest talents?" "Is my job fulfilling and challenging?" I realize that for the majority of Americans the answer to these questions is no. Unfortunately, there is a significant physiological price to be paid for not loving your work. In a recent study on the risk factors for heart disease conducted by the Massachusetts Department of Health, the two greatest risks lie in one's self-happiness rating and level of job satisfaction. Low scores on these two were shown to be better indicators of the likelihood for developing heart disease than high cholesterol, high blood pressure, overweight, and a sedentary lifestyle. The findings were further dramatized by the astounding statistic that more people died of heart attacks on Monday mornings around 9:00 than at any other time of the week! What a powerful demonstration of the mind-body connection.

Why, then, do so many of us continue to risk our lives and quality of life working in jobs that we dislike? The beliefs that are most often responsible are "I have no choice; I need the money"; "I'll never be able to make any money doing what I love to do"; or "I have no idea what I'd enjoy doing or what my greatest talents are." Every one of us has been blessed with at least one God-given gift. For most of us there is at least one activity that we enjoy doing or that we do quite well. *That* is where you begin to investigate what your gifts are.

Arnold Patent, in his book *You Can Have It All*, describes the universal principles that apply to obtaining one's life goals. He also suggests an exercise for identifying talents. It is as follows:

> Make a list of the things you love to do. Limit the list to those activities that create an excitement in you at the mere thought of them. The shorter the list, the easier it is to reach the desired result. Select the item on the list that is most important to you. Do this no matter how much you may resist picking one item. Remember, picking one does not mean you have to give up the others forever. Make a list of the ways you can express the talent you just selected. It is best to do this daily. Keep a separate book for this exercise. Write down every idea that occurs to you, no matter how silly or meaningless it may

seem. The purpose of the exercise is to stimulate your creative mind. After doing the exercise for a period of time, you will have developed a habit pattern that will continually produce creative ways to express what you love to do. The number of ways you can express yourself by doing what you love has no limit.

Scientists' belief that human beings make use of only a small fraction (about 5 to 10 percent) of their brain power lends credence to the statement that your capabilities are limitless. You need only acknowledge that you are seeking a greater level of fulfillment, are willing to change, are ready to take a risk (it could well be a greater risk not to), and will begin the exploration that will lead you to work that you love doing. What a wonderful treat to give to yourself!

MENTAL IMAGERY

This technique of visualization is one that each of us uses every day, but most of the time subconsciously. Our inner dialogue and the messages we continually give ourselves are very often accompanied by inner pictures. In a sense, these images are "waking dreams." Since the 1970s there has been a growing interest within the medical and other health professions in harnessing these images to be used as a conscious therapy. From the pioneering work of O. Carl Simonton, M.D., an oncologist working with cancer patients, to the experiences of ordinary physicians who have made mental imagery an integral part of their treatment, the results have been truly astounding. Even more exciting is the fact that the technique easily lends itself to self-healing, as long as you are willing to practice.

Martin Rossman, M.D., of the University of California Medical Center in San Francisco, and author of *Healing Yourself: A Step-by-Step Program for Better Health Through Im-*

agery, believes that imagery can lead to relief in 90 percent of the problems people bring to their primary care physician. From minor ailments such as back pain, neck pain, arthritis, palpitations, dizziness, and fatigue to conditions as serious as cancer and heart disease, patients can use imagery to address the mental and emotional aspects of their illnesses, thereby helping the physical healing.

I first became aware of mental imagery after hearing on a television talk show about a nine-year-old boy who had healed his inoperable cancerous brain tumor. He had spent about fifteen to twenty minutes daily sitting quietly with his eyes closed, while picturing missiles being fired into his tumor. The remission of his cancer was documented with brain scans. The description of this technique certainly captured my attention.

Shortly thereafter, I came down with yet another sinus infection. I decided to try mental imagery in addition to my usual regimen for the treatment of acute sinusitis. Without having received any formal training in the method, I sat in a straight-backed chair and focused on deep, relaxed breathing for about twenty minutes. The following vision appeared to me. I saw a large sphere completely covered with a slimy, moldy, greenish-gray crud—terrible-looking stuff! At the top of this globe (if you picture the earth, this would be the North Pole) were a group of ten little workmen, clothed in overalls and caps, each holding a high-powered hose and a long-handled push broom. I watched as they methodically began to work their way down the sides of this sphere, hosing and sweeping away the green slime. Underneath was revealed the brightest and healthiest-looking orange I had ever seen. After the orange was completely uncovered, I got up from my chair and at that moment felt the largest clump of postnasal mucus I'd ever had in the back of my throat. As I marveled at the size of the greenish-yellow mass I had then spit into the sink, I could sense that my sinus infection was almost completely resolved. I have never had another since. Needless to say, I remain impressed with the power of mental imagery to treat physical ailments, although it is not the only therapy I used to cure my sinus disease. Another image you can use preventively for sinuses is to begin each day seeing yourself surrounded by several layers of bright, multicolored light. This light can act as a protective shield or as your own personal air filter removing air pollutants before they can enter your nose and sinuses. A very handy image indeed, especially in badly polluted environments.

Mental imagery can also be employed to help you feel more relaxed and peaceful, develop your creative talents, create more fulfillment in relationships, reach your career goals (the clarity of a goal is definitely enhanced when you picture it on a regular basis), and dissolve negative habit patterns. To learn this technique, I recommend Dr. Rossman's book; *Healing Visualizations: Creating Health Through Imagery* by Gerald Epstein, M.D., a professor of psychiatry at Mt. Sinai Medical Center in New York; and *Creative Visualization* by Shakti Gawain, an extraordinary teacher of holistic health.

OPTIMISM AND HUMOR

It may come as a surprise to learn that an optimistic outlook and a good, hearty laugh are beneficial not only mentally but physically. In the research for their book *Healthy Pleasures*, Robert Ornstein, Ph.D., and David Sobel, M.D., found that the healthiest people are optimistic and happy and seem to feel that things will work out no matter what their difficulties. As Ornstein and Sobel put it, "The way they live and envision their lives nourishes their life itself. They expect good things of the world. They expect that their world will be orderly; they expect that other people will like and respect them; and most important, they expect pleasure in much of what they do."

Many of these people maintain a vital sense of humor about life and enjoy a good laugh, more often than not at their own expense. Studies have shown that laughter can improve the function of the immune system. Hearty laughter can be considered a gentle exercise of the body, a form of "inner jogging." Ornstein and Sobel describe the physical effects of laughter:

> A robust laugh gives the muscles of your face, shoulders, diaphragm, and abdomen a good workout. With convulsive or side-splitting laughter, even your arm and leg muscles come into play. Your heart rate and blood pressure temporarily rise, breathing becomes faster and deeper, and oxygen surges through your bloodstream. A vigorous laugh can burn up as many calories per hour as brisk walking or cycling. . . . The afterglow of a hearty laugh is positively relaxing. Blood pressure may temporarily fall, your muscles go limp, and you bask in a mellow euphoria. Some researchers speculate that laughter triggers the release of endorphins, the brain's own opiates; this may account for the pain relief and euphoria that accompany laughter.

Some believe that it is possible to treat disease through laughter. The Gesundheit Institute in Arlington, Virginia, founded and directed by Patch Adams, M.D., focuses on the healing potential of humor. Norman Cousins, in his best-seller *Anatomy of an Illness*, attributed his recovery from ankylosing spondylitis (a potentially crippling arthritic condition) to the many hours he spent watching Marx Brothers movies and reruns of the television show "Candid Camera."

There is some evidence that laughter strengthens the immune system. In one study, research subjects watching a videotape of the comedian Richard Pryor temporarily produced in their saliva elevated levels of antibodies that help combat infections such as colds. Interestingly, the subjects who said they frequently used humor to cope with life stress had consistently higher baseline levels of those protective antibodies.

As Ornstein and Sobel express it, "Laughter is an affirmation of our humanness and an effective antidote to adversity. It can free us to detach and consider problems along new, creative lines. Laughter is a celebration of the unconventional, the unusual, the irregular, the indecorous, the illogical, the nonsensical." The only side effect to this powerful medicine is pleasure. When the question posed to octogenarians is "If you had your life to live over again, what would you do differently?" the answer often is "I'd take life much less seriously." Comedian George Burns, at 95 years of age, has just written the book *Wisdom of the 90s*. He attributes his ability to laugh at himself as well as loving what he does for a living as the most important factors in his longevity.

If you are interested in learning a more pleasurable approach to the entire spectrum of holistic health, *Healthy Pleasures* is an excellent resource.

FORGIVENESS

There might not be a concept more important to mental fitness than that of forgiveness. How often have you thought to yourself, "I am my own worst enemy," or "I sure do make things hard on myself"? Or do you often find yourself blaming someone else for your own problems or stress? The next time you are aware of blaming others, physically point your index finger at them (or preferably their images) and take a look at where the other three curled fingers of that hand are pointed. Forgiveness begins with accepting responsibility for the role you play in shaping your life's experiences. You cannot practice forgiveness on anyone else before starting on yourself. The affirmations "I am always doing the best I can" and "I acknowledge and accept that I am the creative power in my world" are both helpful in learning to forgive yourself.

Stephen Levine, in his book *Healing into Life and Death*, devotes an excellent chapter to forgiveness. It begins with the following sentence: "The beginning of the path of healing is the end of life unlived." It also contains a forgiveness meditation that I often recommend to my patients.

Albert Ellis, Ph.D., a psychologist and founder of the Institute for Rational-Emotive Therapy in New York City, has probably done more psychotherapy sessions than any other psychologist: some 90,000 hours' worth. The following quote of his, from an article by Claire Warga titled "You Are What You Think" in *Psychology Today* (September 1988), helped me better understand the importance of forgiveness in the spectrum of mental health. Ellis said, "My psychotherapeutic philosophy holds that the vast majority of humans, in every part of the world, are much more disturbed than they have to be because they simply will not accept themselves as fallible, incessantly error-prone humans."

You can learn a great deal about forgiveness by watching or (preferably) playing sports. Imagine, for example, a tennis player in an important match. Suppose he misses a shot he thinks he should have made. His response can run the gamut from mild disappointment, as evidenced by a facial expression, to obvious rage, with loud self-berating and racket-throwing. In order to continue to play at an optimal level of performance and remain competitive, he must be able to very quickly forgive himself for having made this bad shot (mistake), since he will have to attempt many more shots in rapid succession. If he continues to hold onto his anger or his belief that he's a bad player for having made a mistake, he will soon lose his confidence, his ability to concentrate, and the match.

This same type of scenario occurs for most of us on a daily basis, although usually not in the sports arena. Although we might have more time than the tennis player to recover from our mistakes, unless we forgive ourselves and let go of the past, we will lose some degree of confidence, the ability to focus and stay in the present, and the capacity to do as well as we know we are capable of doing.

How, then, does the commonly held belief "I know I did not do as well as I am capable of doing" correlate with the affirmation "I am always doing the best I can"? Given all of the circumstances of your life—where and how you were raised, your level of education and training, and the present conditions of your personal life and current level of stress—at every moment of every day, you and I and everyone else are always doing the best we can. That is my belief. To me it feels much better than the alternative, and as you practice it on yourself you will be forgiving others at the same time.

For many high achievers, a capacity for forgiveness has been a critical factor in their success. In order to grow, learn, expand your horizons, and find greater fulfillment in life, you must be willing to change, take risks, and try something new. This cannot be done without making "mistakes," which can also be looked upon as opportunities to learn (just as Bernie Siegel felt illness could be seen as a source of growth). By taking risks you provide yourself an excellent opportunity to practice self-forgiveness. As with anything else, the more you practice, the better you become. "I am always doing the best I can" is not a belief that precludes trying to do better. It allows you the chance to do just that, by helping you to stay in the game, without destroying your self-confidence. It also makes risk-taking and life in general much more fun. If it feels right to you, why not choose this belief? While you're at it, you can add the corollary, "There are no mistakes; only lessons."

MENTAL HEALTH RECOMMENDATIONS: A SUMMARY

Beliefs and affirmations: Identify negative beliefs you would like to change and put your responses into the form of affirmations. Some that are almost always helpful are the following:

> I am always doing the best I can.
> I love and approve of myself.
> Everything is happening in perfect time.
> I love my body.

For chronic sinusitis, add the following:

> My sinuses are now completely healed.
> I declare peace and harmony are within me and surround me at all times.

- *Goals:* Make a list of your goals, desires, and objectives in every realm of holistic health (physical, mental, emotional, spiritual, and social), as long as you believe that they are even remotely possible. Put them into the form of affirmations and add them to your other affirmations to form a composite list. Repeat these regularly either orally or in writing, or record them on a cassette and play them back daily (although listening is not quite as effective as speaking or writing).
- *Choice:* Recognize that you are a unique individual and can choose your own beliefs based on your intuition or whatever feels right for you. Choose to accept your chronic illness as an opportunity for psychological growth, redirection, and ultimately greater enjoyment of your life.

- Desire, belief, and expectation: These will help you achieve any goal. Optimism (the expectation that things will work out well) is also an ingredient found in most healthy people.
- *NLP:* This helps to change beliefs and attitudes, and is a method for excelling in any endeavor (e.g., business, sports, or the creative or performing arts). It should be learned from a certified NLP practitioner. To excel in anything can improve your self-esteem.
- *Work:* Find a job that you love doing and that employs your unique talents. Avoid work environments with especially unhealthy air. Do the Arnold Patent exercise described in this chapter.
- *Humor:* Look for more humor and opportunities for laughter in your life. Lighten up; take life less seriously.
- *Forgiveness:* Remember that you are a human being with imperfections, weaknesses, and flaws, as is everyone else. Learn to accept your mistakes and avoid blaming others. Affirmations can help with this.
- A good friend of mine recites the following poem, "Thinking," every night together with his two young sons, just before putting them to bed:

If you think you are beaten, you are.
If you think you dare not, you don't.
If you like to win, but you think you can't,
It is almost certain you won't.

If you think you'll lose, you're lost,
For out in the world we find,
Success begins with a fellow's will—
It's all in the state of mind.

If you think you are outclassed, you are,
You've got to think high to rise,
You've got to be sure of yourself before
You can ever win a prize.

Life's battles don't always go
To the stronger or faster man,
But soon or late the man who wins
Is the one WHO THINKS HE CAN!

WALTER D. WINTLE

12 EMOTIONAL HEALTH

The emotionally fit are aware of their feelings and are able to express them. I have heard contemporary American culture referred to as the "no-feeling" society. The feelings are certainly present, but as a result of our lifestyle we have constructed such formidable protective barriers around ourselves that to a great extent we have become unconscious of our feelings.

There appear to be only two basic human emotions: love and fear. The so-called negative emotions, such as anger, anxiety, depression, envy, guilt, hatred, hostility, jealousy, loneliness, shame, and worry, are all expressions of fear. The feelings of acceptance, intimacy, joy, and peacefulness are all aspects of love. The greater our degree of fear, the less capable we are of experiencing love.

In our culture it is not socially acceptable to express most of the negative emotions, and men especially are not supposed to show signs of weakness or insecurity or to cry ("Big boys don't cry"). The majority of us have learned to repress these feelings until we are unaware that we even have them. Society has helped us suppress our painful (negative) feelings by perpetuating the myth of an emotionally pain-free existence. The numerous ads in the media for analgesics to treat tension headaches and the common use of alcohol or drugs to dull the pain of an awkward social situation or personal crisis give us the relentless message that not only is pain a bad thing, but that life can be pain free.

If we spent less time avoiding emotional pain, but instead focused our attention on it, accepted it, and relaxed into it, the pain would diminish or even disappear. If we continue to ignore and repress it, it often manifests itself as physical pain, illness, or disease. In fact, chronic sinusitis is usually associated with a tremendous amount of unexpressed anger.

Clyde Reid is director of the Center for New Beginnings in Denver. In his insightful book *Celebrate the Temporary*, he says, "Leaning into life's pain can also be a lifestyle, and is far more satisfying than the avoidance style. It requires small doses of plain courage to look pain in the eye, but it prepares you for more serious pain when it comes. In the meantime, all the energy expended to avoid pain is now available for the business of living."

I am not advocating that you seek out painful experiences, nor am I proposing that you endure prolonged or persistent pain. That is called suffering. Health and happiness do not have prerequisites that require you to suffer. Life is to be enjoyed, but the notion that it can be lived entirely without painful feelings is an unhealthy belief. Pain and joy are intertwined, and the more you allow yourself to accept, embrace, and feel pain, the greater will be your sense of emotional health.

MENTAL/EMOTIONAL OVERLAP

Although mental health focuses primarily on thoughts, beliefs, attitudes, and imagery, and emotional health on feelings, they are for the most part inextricably related. For that matter, all of the aspects of "mind"—mental, emotional, spiritual, and social—are so interrelated that improvement in one area will often have positive ramifications in the others. I have dealt with them separately to enable you to better grasp the scope of each aspect of health and to make it easier to work on each one.

Of the mental-emotional connection, Albert Ellis has said that "virtually all 'emotionally disturbed' individuals actually think crookedly, magically, dogmatically, and unrealistically." David D. Burns, M.D., is the director of the Behavioral Science Research Foundation and acting chairman of psychiatry at the Presbyterian Medical Center of Philadelphia. In *The Feeling Good Handbook: Using the New Mood Therapy in Everyday Life,* he writes:

> Certain kinds of negative thoughts make people unhappy. In fact, I believe that unhealthy, negative emotions—depression, anxiety, excessive anger, inappropriate guilt, etc.—are *always* caused by illogical, distorted thoughts, even if those thoughts may seem absolutely valid at the time. By learning to look at things more realistically, by getting rid of your distorted thinking patterns, you can break out of a bad mood, often in a short period of time, without having to rely on medication or prolonged psychotherapy.

Burns offers the following list of thought distortions:

- All-or-nothing thinking. You classify things into absolute, black-and-white categories.
- Overgeneralization. You view a single negative situation as a never-ending pattern of defeat.
- Mental filtering. You dwell on negatives and overlook positives.
- Discounting the positive. You insist your accomplishments or positive qualities "don't count."
- Magnification or minimization. You blow things out of proportion or shrink their importance inappropriately.

- Making "should" statements. You criticize yourself and others by using the terms *should, shouldn't, must, ought,* and *have to.*
- Emotional reasoning. You reason from how you feel. If you feel like an idiot, you assume you must be one. If you don't feel like doing something, you put it off.
- Jumping to conclusions. You "mind read," assuming, without definite evidence of it, that people are reacting negatively to you. Or you "fortune tell," arbitrarily predicting bad outcomes.
- Labeling. You identify with your shortcomings. Instead of saying, "I made a mistake," you tell yourself, "I'm such a jerk . . . a real loser."
- Personalization and blame. You blame yourself for something you weren't entirely responsible for, or you blame others and ignore the impact of your own attitudes or behavior.

It is now widely accepted that negative thoughts and the feelings they engender contribute to physical illness. Conversely, recent research has revealed that positive emotions cause the body to produce substances that are identical to the ingredients in pharmaceutical drugs that help people feel better. For example, when you feel peace and tranquility, your body makes molecules identical to those in the tranquilizer Valium. When you feel exhilarated, your body produces interleuken-2—in its pharmaceutical form, a powerful anticancer drug, each dose of which costs nearly $40,000. If you were to engage in an especially fun-filled activity, your body might make millions of dollars' worth of interleuken-2.

PSYCHOTHERAPY

Traditional psychotherapy based on Freudian principles has been the conventional approach to the treatment of mental and emotional disorders. Like traditional medicine, this is a disease-oriented approach, in which patients come to be fixed. Still, psychiatrists, psychoanalysts, and psychotherapists might have distinctly different ways of treating the same problem.

Today, the majority of patients who see psychiatrists are labeled with a psychiatric diagnosis and treated with psychotherapeutic drugs. The arsenal of these drugs is constantly expanding as researchers explore the physiology of the human brain. In fact, Prozac, one of the newest antidepressants, has quickly risen almost to the top of the list of most prescribed drugs in this country. Psychiatry is definitely moving in the direction of less counseling and more drug therapy, although every one of these drugs has potentially unpleasant side effects. The emphasis is on treating the symptom with drugs rather than encouraging the patient to change attitudes or behavior, or just to be with their pain and learn from it.

A new wrinkle in psychotherapy is the rapidly expanding field of cognitive therapy. Therapist and theorist Albert Ellis has pioneered a psychotherapy that stresses the importance of cognitions—ideas, beliefs, assumptions, interpretations, and thinking processes—in the origins and treatment of emotional disturbance. There are many different types of cognitive therapies, all of which teach people how to evaluate critically their own thought processes and to trust in their own reasoning ability, rather than adhere to the standards and norms of others. These theories are based on the power of people to transform their current beliefs. Unlike the Freudian approach, the focus is not on the past but on the present: *If you can change what you think, you'll change the way you feel.* In a society that looks for fast solutions, this brief form of psychotherapy usually takes under a year, much less time than the traditional psychotherapeutic approach.

Increasingly, the job of counseling is being assumed by psychologists, social workers, pastoral counselors, and anyone else with a counseling degree. The health care industry, particularly the medical insurance companies, have helped to create these changes. They have discouraged long-term psychotherapy by reimbursing for a limited number of visits to the therapist; by paying for only a portion of the fee, with a large copayment assumed by the patient; or by not paying for this service at all.

Although this book is intended to be a self-help guide, and holistic medicine focuses on self-healing, I strongly advocate psychotherapy as an important means of improving your health. In addition to the obvious mental and emotional benefits, physical effects have now also been documented. Norman Cousins conducted a study at the UCLA School of Medicine that involved two groups of cancer patients. The group that had psychotherapy for one and a half hours a week for six weeks showed profound positive changes in their immune systems. The group that received no counseling had no change in immune function.

More and more therapists are becoming aware of the connection between psychotherapy and spiritual growth, and have incorporated spirituality into their therapeutic program. I encourage you to seek a therapist who has made this transition and who understands and appreciates the importance of spirituality in the healing process. I would also recommend someone who practices cognitive therapy. The therapist should be someone with whom you feel comfortable. It would be prudent to interview several before selecting one.

Goals are extremely important. Try to clarify what it is you want from psychotherapy. Be as specific as possible. The greater your clarity, the shorter your therapy. However, you might be in such emotional pain that drug therapy sounds very good to you, and that might be just what you need. Find a psychiatrist and get started. You also have the option of seeing a holistic physician. It should be apparent from this text that psychotherapy is one aspect of such a physician's job.

There are times when the symptoms of disease—

whether physical or mental—can be so overwhelming that people feel paralyzed or suicidal. Life seems to be at a standstill and they feel worthless and are without hope. You must determine your own threshold of discomfort. When it has been reached, seek help in a way that feels best to you. This is your program, and no one knows you better than you do. To achieve a balanced state of holistic health, you cannot allow yourself to get stuck in one area for too long. Try to learn something from each experience, and then move on. In some instances, this can take a year or more. Whether you are suffering from the death of a loved one, a divorce, a business failure, or a chronic or terminal disease, you must go through a period of grieving and adjust to your loss. Elisabeth Kübler-Ross, M.D., a psychiatrist and author of the classic text *On Death and Dying*, has identified five stages in this process: denial, anger, bargaining, depression, and then acceptance. Allow yourself to feel all of your feelings, and know that there is something to be gained from them. Realize that however miserable you feel, it is only temporary. Remember that to live without pain is to live an incomplete life.

MEDITATION AND BREATHING THERAPY

As a society, I believe we do not allow ourselves to feel, but how do we manage to avoid our feelings? Workaholism might be the most common means of escape. Our minds are so busy with important thoughts that there is neither room nor time for feelings. Another means of escape, drug abuse, has become such a threat to our culture's stability that our government has declared a war on drugs. That's fine, but it is only another example of symptomatic treatment. With all the publicity and billions of dollars being spent on this campaign, I have never heard any drug enforcement official question why so many millions of people have risked their lives to avoid confronting their feelings. Our extremely fast-paced society and its quick-fix syndrome are other symptoms of avoidance; we are eager for fast and easy ways to satisfy our needs for food, sex, money, energy, entertainment, exercise, transportation, communication, and health.

Why the hurry? Where are we running? The quest for money, power, material wealth, recognition, and intellectual superiority have become major distractions and, in many instances, addictions. Life could be infinitely more enjoyable and enriching if we would just slow down! We can smell the roses or simply tune in to life—to the messages our bodies are always giving us, to what we are thinking and feeling, to the value of our relationships, and to our connection to the earth and to our fellow human beings.

One way to slow down is to learn to breathe more consciously. For most of us, breathing is an unconscious process that begins traumatically at birth. After that, little attention is paid to breathing other than the ability to keep on doing it. The medical profession has not been curious as to how humans can improve this unconscious function by doing it more efficiently and consciously.

Meditation is one of several disciplines that can be described as conscious breathing. Meditation has several benefits. It slows you down and allows you to inhale more oxygen, which is, after all, the most critical nutrient for human health. Meditation is relaxing (it is an integral part of most stress management programs) and keeps you focused on the present, not allowing you to hang onto past regrets or worries about the future. It can empty your mind of thoughts and, if practiced enough, can help to bring more feelings to the surface, allow creative ideas to flow, and heighten spiritual awareness. It is also quite effective in lowering high blood pressure, slowing the heart rate, reducing pain (especially headaches), and is an adjunct in treating heart disease and many other physical ailments. Former Harvard researcher Charles Alexander, Ph.D., taught transcendental meditation to a group of nursing-home patients. In 1990, he reported that over a three-year period, all the meditators survived, compared with only 62.6 of the nonmeditators.

Ideally, meditation should be practiced in a quiet place. Sit on the floor cross-legged or in a chair with your feet on the floor and your back unsupported. Abdominal breathing should be done through your nose at a rate of approximately three full breaths (inhale and exhale) per minute. To practice, place a hand on your belly: In abdominal breathing, your abdomen will protrude with each inhalation and flatten with each exhalation. To stay focused on the breath and avoid being distracted by your thoughts (they will be there, but just let them come and go), it helps to repeat silently a very short affirmation or just one word, such as *love, peace,* or whatever you'd like, on both inhalation and exhalation. At first try doing it for five minutes a day, then gradually increase the time to twenty minutes twice a day. Another technique you could try is to count slowly and silently to five ("one thousand one, one thousand two," etc.) on the inhalation, hold your breath for a count of five, exhale for five, then pause for five before beginning the next cycle. Don't be discouraged if this feels difficult at first. Sitting and breathing without thinking, listening to music, or obviously accomplishing something is not easy for most Americans. I can assure you, though, that if you continue to practice, you will soon begin to appreciate the many benefits of this simple routine. The next time you feel especially stressed, pay attention to the way you are breathing. You will probably find that your breaths are shallow and irregular; many people even hold their breath when they're anxious. This would be an ideal time to give a five-minute meditation a try. Meditation can also be a good way to start the day (it's energizing in the morning) and as a means of unwinding after work or before bed (it's relaxing later in the day). Books on meditation are widely available. One that I would recommend is *A Gradual Awakening* by Stephen Levine.

Yoga is another discipline of conscious breathing combined with movement. One of the asanas (yogic exercises), called the lion, is especially effective in helping the sinuses to drain. It relaxes facial muscles and in so doing, the ostia open and sinus pressure can be relieved. According to Mardi Erdmann, a noted yoga instructor and author of *Undercover Exercise*, the lion is performed in the following manner: sit with your hands (palms down) on your thighs and your eyes closed; take a deep breath through your nose, your face quiet and relaxed but poised for action. On the exhale, open your eyes and mouth wide, stick your tongue way out (down to your chin), extend your hands and arms straight out in front of you with your fingers extended wide; your breath is forced out of your mouth over the tongue with an accompanying air sound (*not* a voice sound).

There are many varieties of breath therapy, sometimes referred to as "breath work." What they have in common is the ability to make you more aware of deeply held and often painful feelings. Breath therapies are similar to meditation in that they use the focus on breath to empty the mind of thoughts, but they differ in the style of breathing. Most breath therapies use the technique of connected breathing, which is much more rapid than the breathing of meditation. Each inhalation immediately follows the exhalation of the preceding breath. Mouth breathing is usually recommended, and both abdominal and chest breathing are used. The therapy can be performed even more effectively under water with the use of a snorkel. Two of the more popular breath therapies are rebirthing and holotropic therapy, in which loud music accompanies the breathing. I would suggest attempting breath work only under the direction of a skilled breath therapist. Because of the emotional release that results from this work, these experts often include psychotherapy as a part of the process. The therapist I have worked with is supervised by a psychiatrist. Although the field is still in its infancy, breath therapy is being recognized as a powerful tool for emotional health.

DREAMS AND JOURNALING

"Dreams are extraordinarily reliable commentaries on the life you really live—the people you care about, the events you anticipate, the problems you are trying to solve," says Robert Langs, M.D., a psychoanalyst and chief of the Center for Communicative Research at Beth Israel Hospital in New York City. "Every dream reflects an unconscious response to an emotionally charged situation in waking reality. [Dreams] consistently point out aspects of your feelings that you have overlooked, ignored, or tried to keep at bay. My own studies have indicated that the very process of remembering a dream promotes emotional stability. Analyzing dreams is an extremely helpful way of maintaining your equilibrium and your emotional balance."

There are at least two obstacles that prevent us from using our dreams as tools for better emotional health. First, most dreams are quickly forgotten. Second, the few that we do remember are filled with symbolism and imagery that do not lend themselves to simple interpretation. Dr. Langs believes that it is more natural to forget a dream than to remember it, because of our unconscious efforts to protect ourselves from mental and emotional pain. He thinks that we should trust our unconscious intuition. "When the conscious mind is ready to cope with the meanings embedded in a dream," he says, "in most instances you will dream some other version of it later— and remember it."

If you are able to recall dreams and would like to use them in your self-healing process, keep a pad and pencil or a tape recorder by your bed. By writing dreams down or verbally recording them immediately after you awaken, you will retain more of the details. The more often you do this, the better you may be able to understand the symbolism of your dreams. There are psychotherapists, usually with a Jungian orientation, who are skilled in dream interpretation and can help you. Three books I recommend are: *Do You Dream?* by Tony Crisp, which offers many alternative interpretations of symbols; *The Dictionary of Symbols* by J. E. Cirlot; and *What Your Dreams Teach You* by Alex Lukeman. A dream, however, is highly personal and, ultimately, the dreamer is the only one who can appreciate its deepest meanings.

Journaling is the keeping of a written record of your feelings, thoughts, and any other information you'd like to clarify for yourself. If journaling is done on a regular basis it can increase self-knowledge and be both enlightening and enlivening. In a sense you become your own therapist or your own best friend; instead of trying to convey what you're feeling to another person, you're telling it to yourself. Communicating with yourself this way seems to allow for greater clarity and ease, probably because there is much less concern about judgment—you are the only one who will be reading what you write, and you don't have to worry about spelling or grammar. In the book *Opening Up*, James W. Pennebaker, Ph.D., documents the benefits to one's physical health that can be gained by writing about upsetting or traumatic experiences. If you write on a regular basis, your journal becomes an emotional "diary."

EMOTIONAL RELEASE

The two most recognized emotional ailments are anxiety and depression. I have found anger to be a component of both, but especially the latter. In fact, many psychiatrists believe that repressed anger is the "fuel" for depression. Although it is not always apparent to my patients, it has become clear to me that anger is almost universally present both as a cause and as a feeling that helps to maintain chronic sinusitis.

Anger is a perfectly normal human emotion. We usually feel some degree of anger on a daily basis. But anger has been stigmatized, and its expression is usually unacceptable. Much of the negative attitude toward anger has to do with fears about how this strong feeling will affect or be perceived by others. We're often afraid that our anger will hurt someone else, or that we may be perceived as harsh, abrasive, offensive, cruel, or even emotionally unstable. Comments such as "He's in a rage," "She really flew off the handle," or "Don't go near him, he's having a fit" help to reinforce our fear of expressing anger. Much of the time we repress it so quickly and unconsciously that we may not even know that we are mad. I have seen many patients who have had this conditioned response since early childhood, and are so adept that they are unaware of what they have been doing.

The medical profession has endorsed psychotherapy as the best means to deal with "excessive" anger and fear (i.e., depression and anxiety, along with a host of other emotional disorders). The traditional vehicles for treating these conditions are drug therapy and counseling. Both are mental or mind-focused tools. Drugs affect the brain directly, and most psychotherapy is a verbal and intellectual exercise that may take years to complete.

In recent years some psychotherapists have begun teaching their clients methods of using sound or their own bodies to quickly and effectively release anger. Not surprisingly, the most common of these techniques is screaming. It certainly worked well when we were young kids. The most difficult problem with screaming is finding a place where you won't attract attention or be considered crazy. Doing it in the basement of your home, in a closet, or in the car with the windows rolled up are all possibilities. If you want to make less noise you can hold your hands over your mouth when you scream. Take a deep abdominal breath just before screaming, and try to bring up the sound from your diaphragm or deep in your chest, and not from your throat, in order to protect your vocal cords. Slowly move your upper body or trunk from side to side and up and down while you're screaming (this will be a real challenge if you're sitting in your car). Two or three screams in succession are enough.

Punching is another effective method for venting anger. I have a heavy punching bag and boxing gloves, and I make daily visits to the basement for just a couple of minutes of punching. I do this preventively rather than waiting until I'm in a rage. However, when I do feel a lot of anger, punching is a great way to release it. Instead of a punching bag, you can also hit or punch pillows or your sofa, using your fists or a baseball bat or broomstick.

If you have young children, the Yogi Bear Bop Bag may help you teach the same technique. A gift of this toy shows that you accept and approve of your children's anger. You can encourage them to pretend that the Bop Bag is either you or their brother or sister or whoever it is they are angry at. A friend of mine has done this with his children and it works quite well. What a gift of emotional health to give your kids—to let them know that it's OK to be angry and to provide them with an acceptable means of expressing it.

Another technique involves stamping the floor with your right foot (first raise your knee waist high) while simultaneously bringing your right arm across your chest, elbow bent, and then forcefully bringing it back to its original position just as your foot hits the floor. This movement is accompanied by a grunt. Then repeat the same thing on the left side. Continue alternating sides for three to four minutes. When you've finished you'll feel a bit tired but much more relaxed.

I had one patient who interrupted as I began explaining anger release and said, "I don't have a problem with that. I go to a discount store and buy some cheap glasses, and whenever I get really angry I throw them against a brick wall and feel much better."

If none of these physical methods interests you, then try talking to yourself or expressing your anger to your spouse, another family member, close friend, or directly to the person with whom you are angry. Whatever feels comfortable to you is fine, but choose *something* and try it. Anger release has been extremely helpful for sinus sufferers.

Screaming is not the only method of emotional release left behind in early childhood. For men especially, crying is a luxury that is seldom indulged. In our society men cry only one-fifth as often as women do. Somewhere are "oceans" of tears that Americans have not allowed themselves to shed. Yet recent evidence from tear researcher William Frey suggests that the tears produced by emotional crying, as opposed to those triggered by injury or physical pain, may help the body release stress and dispose of toxic substances. Tears also contain endorphins, the adrenal hormone ACTH, the ovarian hormone prolactin (in women's tears only), and growth hormones, all of which are released by stress.

The vast majority of people report that crying improves mood and offers a welcome release of tensions. At least one study of men and women with peptic ulcers or colitis showed that they were less likely to cry compared to their healthy peers. These patients were more likely to regard crying as a sign of weakness or loss of control. It may not be easy at first, but if you feel the tears coming, let go and allow them to flow. Crying is a healthy thing to do, both physically and emotionally.

PLAY

Play is another thing that many of us have relegated to childhood. As a means of expressing joy, passion, exhilaration, and at times even ecstasy, play is an essential component of emotional health. The notion that play is something to be abandoned as soon as you grow up and get a job is an unhealthy belief. In fact, if you've found a job that you love doing, then work and play can become almost indistinguishable. As George Halas, former owner of the Chicago Bears football team, once said, "It's only work if there's someplace else you'd rather be."

Whether or not you've been able to experience work as play, I suggest that you find at least one activity other than work that you thoroughly enjoy. America is a recreational paradise. Even so, there are still many adults who have never given themselves the opportunity to play. Few public schools do an adequate job of teaching this secondary skill. Some private schools, which require participation in sports and strongly encourage involvement in theater, art, and music, are much better in this respect. Boy Scouts and Girl Scouts are good, although play isn't their primary focus, and most summer camps are even better.

I recommend either sports, games, dance, and other activities requiring some body movement, or active creative pursuits such as playing a musical instrument, acting, singing, painting, crafts, or gardening. Although I realize that many people derive great pleasure from playing cards or chess and other board games and from collecting stamps, say, or coins, all these are mental exercises. In our society, we already spend most of our time exercising our minds. To create a healthier balance, we should be looking for activities that utilize our bodies, allow us to better express our feelings and creativity, and perhaps even bring us to a greater level of spiritual attunement. Ideally the activity should be something so consuming and absorbing that it requires total attention. In that way it provides a pleasurable escape from our normal tension and stress and habitual thoughts.

If you played little as a child, or never developed a hobby

or strong interest in any particular recreational activity, choose something that instinctively appeals to you. Then find a good teacher or a class and learn the basics. Be prepared to make mistakes and look silly. That's part of the risk of doing something new. After that first step (always the most difficult one), it will be a matter of making a commitment and practicing. The better you become, the more you'll enjoy and appreciate the benefits of the activity. If you are not interested in learning something new, I suggest a simple activity such as walking or hiking. What's important is to choose something and do it on a regular basis, for at least one hour three times a week.

The importance of play cannot be overemphasized. We live in a culture where work has become the greatest addiction; where for many, achievement, accomplishment, and net financial worth determine self-worth. In such an environment, attaining a sense of wholeness and balance requires that we regularly and, for at least a short time, let go of that responsible, mature, working adult and get back in touch with our playful "inner child."

EMOTIONAL HEALTH RECOMMENDATIONS:
A SUMMARY

- Love and fear: These are the two basic human emotions. All other feelings are aspects of these. The more of one you feel, the less you'll feel of the other.
- Mental/emotional overlap: Unhealthy, negative emotions, such as depression and anxiety, are frequently caused by illogical, distorted, and unrealistic thoughts.
- Psychotherapy: Choose a psychotherapist carefully from among a group of mental health professionals that include psychiatrists, psychologists, holistic physicians, social workers, pastoral counselors, and

those with degrees in counseling. Be clear on your objectives before beginning.

- Meditation: This involves conscious breathing, with benefits in every realm of holistic health. Start with five minutes twice a day and gradually increase to twenty minutes.
- Breath therapy: Any one of a number of methods based on conscious breathing may be used. They help uncover deeply held emotions. The method should be learned from a breath therapist.
- Dream interpretation: The very process of remembering a dream promotes emotional stability. Record dreams in writing or with a tape recorder as soon as you awaken.
- Journaling: Keeping a daily written record of your thoughts and feelings will help you to become your own therapist and best friend.
- Emotional release: Practice at least one anger release technique daily. Most are physical methods that include screaming, punching, hitting, and stamping. Crying can improve your mood, release tension, and remove toxins from the body.
- Play: Select a sport, game, activity, or creative pursuit requiring body movement. Try to practice it for one hour three times a week. Allow yourself to become more childlike.
- Remember, *if you can't feel it, you can't heal it.*

13 SPIRITUAL HEALTH

I want to make it clear that this discussion of spiritual health is not a discourse on religion, although it is based on truths common to all religions. To me, spiritual health means a heightened awareness of a power greater than oneself. This power can be referred to as God, the Creator, the Source, Infinite Intelligence, Jesus, Adonai, Yahweh, Allah, or your inner healer, voice, teacher, guide, child, or higher self. Whatever term feels most comfortable to you is the right one. A program of spiritual fitness will balance the metaphysical with the material, giving you more access to this higher power. The result will be a profound reduction in your feelings of fear and an increased capacity to love both yourself and others unconditionally. Additional benefits might include reversing heart disease (spiritual health is an integral part of Dr. Dean Ornish's treatment program) and eliminating substance abuse (spirituality is the basis of the Twelve-Step programs used for alcohol, drug, and other addictions). A spiritual fitness program is also great for healing sick sinuses!

Each of the world's great religions prescribes a method for gaining greater awareness of God, a term I will use because it is the most common. Each religion believes that it is the one correct path to spiritual enlightenment. All of these faiths express their essence in a single moral principle:

> Buddhism: *Hurt not others in ways that you yourself would find hurtful.*   UDANAVARGA 5:18

Christianity: *All things whatsoever you would that men should do to you, do ye even so to them.*
MATTHEW 7:12

Confucianism: *Do not unto others what you would not have them do unto you.* ANALECTS 15:23

Hinduism: *Do naught unto others which would cause you pain if done to you.* MAHABHARATA 5:1517

Islam: *No one of you is a believer until he desires for his brother that which he desires for himself.* SUNAN

Judaism: *Thou shalt love thy neighbor as thyself.*
LEVITICUS 19:18

Judaism: *What is hateful to you, do not to your fellow man.* TALMUD, CHABBAT 31a

An equally important objective of most of these religions is that the believer love God or come to know God. The essence of the Judeo-Christian doctrine is expressed in the words that Jewish people are instructed to repeat twice daily, "You shall love the Lord your God, with all your heart, with all your soul, and with all your might."

What hasn't been quite so clear to most of us is *how* one loves God. Some have found their answer by living in harmony with nature. James Lovelock, Ph.D., in his book *The Ages of Gaia: A Biography of Our Living Earth,* describes our planet and everything on it as a single living organism. He believes that the dynamic forces that have shaped the globe for the past 4.5 billion years are still modifying the environment to allow the survival of all life forms and that this process is guided by an intrinsic homeostatic mechanism. People who live close to the earth recognize this guiding intelligence as God. Its essence is found not only in the earth, but in themselves and every other living organism on the planet. This life force is referred to as chai (pronounced "hi") in Hebrew and qi (pronounced "chee") in Chinese. This life force is the core spiritual component of every human being and our common bond with our Creator, the earth, our fellow human beings, and all other life forms.

For many people in today's urban technological society, however, God is now found in science. These people have lost any sense of proximity or harmony with the earth, along with the awareness that technology is contributing to its destruction. They expect science to provide them with food and water, stimulate their minds, entertain them, allow them to exercise conveniently, solve most urban problems, fix the environmental crisis it has created, and also heal our diseased bodies. However, science is restricted to the material world, one that can only be experienced through our five physical senses: sight, hearing, touch, taste, and smell. Science is the world of effect. Beyond it, in the realm of the metaphysical, lies cause. *Metaphysics*, defined in Webster's *New World Dictionary* as "the branch of philosophy that deals with first principles and seeks to explain the nature of being or reality and the origin and structure of the world," refers to ideas and concepts beyond the scope of our five senses.

Science believes that the universe is ordered and that it obeys the law of cause and effect; e.g., for every action there is an equal and opposite reaction. However, scientific method on its own is incapable of generating new ideas. In *Where Is Science Going?*, physicist Max Planck wrote, "When the pioneer in science sends forth the groping fingers of his thoughts, he must have a vivid, intuitive imagination, for new ideas are not generated by deduction, but by an artistically creative imagination." In the field of health, psychoneuroimmunology, a product of this type of creative thinking, is building a solid scientific bridge between the world of the physical and the world of the metaphysical. I am hoping that this book will enable you to walk across that bridge with me.

Our modern lifestyle has created a distance between humanity and the earth's natural rhythms. Yet our spiritual essence, the divine spark or life energy within each of us, is transcendent and connects us to all of creation. This concept has been repeated throughout history by almost every prophet and spiritual teacher of every religion. Jesus put it most succinctly: "The kingdom of God is within." I believe that in contemporary society the simplest and most effective way to learn to love God is to learn to love yourself.

The "self" I am referring to is not exactly the one you have come to know. Many of us spend our lives confusing our traits, habits, and actions with ourselves. "This is who I am," we say. Psychology refers to this sense of self as the ego, our conscious personality. We spend almost all of our waking time in the ego, and it constitutes much of the mental and emotional aspects of the self. However, there is still far more to a human being than these components. W. Brugh Joy, M.D., a pioneer in holistic medicine and the author of *Joy's Way* and *Avalanche—Heretical Reflections on the Dark and the Light*, offers the analogy of the human ego as a subatomic particle on the tip of a hair on the tail of a dog, wagging the dog. An entire person, including the spiritual component, encompasses a great deal more than the human intellect can comprehend. There are, however, many ways to explore these vast realms of your unconscious and discover a much deeper sense of love and appreciation for the unique individual that you really are. This process can result in a greater degree of unconditional love for yourself and others, and in that feeling lies an experience of God or a power greater than yourself. What follows are several methods to assist you on this enlivening journey. To help clarify my own goal of spiritual health, I often repeat to myself this saying by the late Teilhard de Chardin, a former priest: "Joy is the most infallible sign of the presence of God!"

MEANING, PURPOSE, AND INTUITION

If you have ever asked yourself the question, "Who am I?," "Where am I going?," or "What am I here to do?," you have already begun your spiritual journey. These questions often arise spontaneously as a result of a heightened sense of mortality, as with advancing age or with a chronic or terminal disease. But many who seek to better understand the meaning of their lives are neither old nor sick. They might have attained their life's goals, or realized the American Dream, a vision that embraces society's values of financial success, power, and public recognition. Having achieved "all anyone could ever want," they often find it a hollow success. They feel an emptiness that begs the questions: "Is that all there is to life?"; "Now what?"; "Isn't there anything more?" Until now, their life's meaning had been defined by society, a definition that was imposed externally rather than one that came from within.

For me, the answers began to unfold when I encountered the work of Elisabeth Kübler-Ross, M.D. This remarkable psychiatrist has been investigating the phenomena of death and dying for most of her career, perhaps longer than any other member of the medical community. Kubler-Ross has concluded from her many years of research that "death does not exist"! She believes that what we call death is merely the shedding of a physical shell housing an immortal spirit, that our time spent in these bodies on earth is but a very brief part of the total span of our existence, and that to live well while we are here means to learn to love.

Initially I was stunned by her words. This was medical science's leading authority on the one subject that most unnerves physicians—who are trained to equate death with failure—and she was making what sounded like some very unscientific remarks. I was unable to dismiss them, however, and in the seven years since learning of her conclusions, I have confirmed for myself their validity. Believing in the existence of spirit and recognizing love as a means of gaining access to its healing potential have helped me to transform not only my medical practice but my life as well. This perspective has provided me with a new direction, goals, and values; it has reduced dramatically my fear of death and enriched my life beyond measure.

Each of us responds differently. An answer that might inspire a greater sense of meaning and direction for one might do nothing for another. What is most important is that you begin asking the questions. If you have taken that first step, as long as you are patient you'll find what you're looking for. The answers might not come like bolts of lightning, but perhaps like a light controlled by a dimmer switch, gradually illuminating a dark or unexplored aspect of your mind. Your guide along this new path will be your intuition. I have heard this inner voice described as "God talking to you." Your progress on this journey of change will be determined by the degree to which you trust your intuition.

The quiet, subtle messages from your intuition have a tough time competing for your attention. Most of the inner messages you hear come from your ego and are loud, often negative, and based on fear. However, if you learn to listen, you will begin to hear a "still, small voice" from the depths of your awareness. If you are interested in developing your sense of intuition, you will have to slow down, eliminate distractions, and do a lot less talking. Meditation, conscious breathing, and slow, relaxing (not brisk, exercise-oriented) walks are all helpful methods of learning to listen to this inner voice.

Learning to follow your intuition is both a life-changing adventure and an enlivening exercise that strengthens your life energy. Just as with any other type of exercise, practice is required. The more you can follow that "hunch" or "gut instinct" or "deep inner voice" and get results that feel good to you, the more you will trust it. This is the foundation upon which faith is built—faith in oneself, God, and the universe. It can become the basis for the belief that the world is really a safe and loving place, where it is okay to trust. If you can learn to trust your intuition, this trust can then extend to the way you interact with the world and can dramatically reduce the amount of stress in your life. This doesn't mean that you will ignore known risks to your health, safety, and security, but it will offer a means of minimizing fear.

There will be instances in which you believe you have been following your intuition and yet the results are painful. You quit your old job only to find less satisfaction with the new one, you move to a new home that turns out to create a lot more headaches than the one you left, or you divorce a spouse and marry someone else with whom you have similar conflicts. These are not necessarily mistakes. They can be seen as lessons. When we were students and failed to learn a subject, we were given a chance to repeat the course. Life can present lessons to us in much the same way, and often painfully.

If you are questioning the meaning of your life, it can be helpful to look back at some of your most painful experiences. Look at the role you played in each one and how you might have contributed to the situation. Ask yourself if there were recognizable patterns of behavior. For example, I have been treating a patient for chronic back pain, which at times has incapacitated her. Before the first attack, her life was a whirlwind of activity—mother, housewife, PTA, sales job, and aerobics instructor. The back pain made it nearly impossible for her to continue with any of her former responsibilities. As soon as it had subsided, however, she resumed her hectic pace, and within a year the problem had returned. This time it was worse, and it put her out of commission for nearly three months. During this period of inactivity, while lying on her back, she began to understand her overwhelming desire to achieve and her strong need to give to others. Without her achievements or the ability to give, she felt worthless. Like so many Americans, she did not feel entitled to love unless she was accomplishing at a high level or taking care of others. She gave very little to herself. Rather than taking the time to learn and appreciate what it means to be a human being, she had become a human doing, and quite a good one at that. Her back has been much better for nearly a year, and she has developed a lifestyle that is much more gentle, nurturing, and healthy. She gives more to herself, works only part-time, and, as a result, is able to spend more time with her family. From this experience she has developed a much greater degree of trust in her intuition, as it directs her on a path of caring for herself with more compassion. Facing an exceptionally painful situation with forgiveness and acceptance rather than anger and fear will bring greater meaning to your life and give you an opportunity to grow spiritually. *Man's Search for Meaning* by Viktor Frankl, M.D., a survivor of a Nazi concentration camp, is an inspirational book on this subject.

Others find greater meaning by conducting their lives as if they have very little time left to live. In his book on spiritual health, *The Road Less Traveled*, M. Scott Peck, M.D., describes the benefits of living with "death on your left shoulder." This approach quickly and dramatically puts life into a different perspective. It forces you to reexamine your values and decide what is really important.

Whatever route you take, as you look for meaning in life you will usually discover greater purpose. Every individual has at least one unique talent or God-given gift. Often it is in the expression of this gift that one finds purpose. To me, one's purpose is to share his or her gift and, as a result, leave the world a better place. I know of no more effective way to realize your purpose than working on a personalized program of holistic health. Several of my student/patients have realized that their gift is for healing, a discovery that has caused them to redirect their professional careers. Some of life's greatest joys come from practicing your gifts and doing what you love to do. Getting paid for doing it can be an added bonus.

PRAYER

Prayer is both a spiritual exercise and the standard Western form of meditation. A Gallup poll in 1988 found that 88 percent of Americans pray. Most of those who do pray have a greater sense of well-being than those who don't. A majority said that they experience a sense of peace when they pray, have received answers to their prayers, and have felt divinely inspired or "led by God" to perform some specific action. Those who said they felt an experience of the divine during prayer are the people who have the highest rating in general well-being or satisfaction with their lives. More than 70 percent of Americans believe prayer can lead to physical, emotional, or spiritual healing.

In a study conducted by Randolph Byrd, M.D., at the San Francisco General Medical Center, Christians were asked to pray for half of a group of 393 hospitalized heart disease patients; no one was assigned to pray for the other half. The patients were unaware of which group they were in. The results showed that a majority of those who were prayed for needed less medical intervention during their hospital stay than those in the control group.

Herbert Benson, M.D., a Harvard cardiologist, has been conducting research that has conclusively demonstrated that prayer benefits health. He began his research in 1968, using subjects who practiced transcendental meditation. They meditated with a mantra, a single word with no meaning to its user, such as *om*. Dr. Benson found that repetition of the mantra replaced the arousing thoughts that otherwise kept them tense during most waking hours. This resulted in a lower metabolic rate, slower heart rate, lower blood pressure, and slower breathing.

Dr. Benson then studied Christians and Jews who prayed rather than meditated. He asked Roman Catholic subjects to repeat "Hail Mary, full of grace" or "Lord Jesus Christ, have mercy upon me." Jews used "Shalom," the peace greeting, or "Echad," meaning "one." Protestants used the first line of the Lord's Prayer, "Our Father, who art in heaven," or the opening of Psalm 23, "The Lord is my shepherd." The phrases all had the same physiological effect as the meditation. Dr. Benson has found that all major religious traditions use simple repetitive prayers. Such repetitions, his research suggests, create what he calls the relaxation response (RR). This response is the opposite of the stress reaction widely known as the flight-or-fight response: in human beings, the physical reaction to perceived danger.

As he continued his studies, Dr. Benson found that faith affects the physiological benefits of RR and that prayer initiates the response. He also found a connection between RR and exercise: when runners meditated or prayed as they ran, their bodies were more efficient. They were able to achieve even greater efficiency by matching the cadence of their short prayers to the rhythm of their stride.

Since 1988, Dr. Benson and psychologist Jared Kass have been conducting a series of programs at the Mind/Body Medical Institute at Boston's New England Deaconess Hospital. They have invited priests, ministers, and rabbis to investigate the spiritual and health implications of prayer. *They found that people who feel themselves in touch with God are less likely to get sick—and better able to cope when they do.* Drs. Benson and Kass developed a psychological scale for measuring spirituality both before and after prayer. Those high in spirituality, which Benson defines as the feeling that "there is more than just you" and as not necessarily religious, scored high in psychological health. They also have fewer stress-related symptoms. Next, he found that people high in spirituality gain the most from meditation training; they show the greatest rise on a life-purpose index as well as the sharpest drop in pain. The nearly three-quarters of the American population who already believe that prayer can be therapeutic now have additional confirmation: science has shown that as prayer strengthens the spirit, it can also heal the body.

For those of you who already pray, I recommend that you continue. For those who would like to begin, I suggest you start with any prayer with which you might be comfortable or can remember from your religious training. The Lord's Prayer is familiar to most Christians, and the majority of Jews know the Shema and Viahavta. Try to establish a regular routine and repeat the prayer morning and night. You might have a favorite psalm or a passage from the Bible or a prayer book that is especially meaningful. Add it to your daily regimen. I have found three psalms in particular to be especially healing: 121, which I repeat every morning; 91, which I say in late afternoons or after work; and 23, which I say before bed.

In addition to the prayers and psalms associated with religion and the Bible, you might be interested in more personal prayer. To do this, talk to God as if you are speaking to your best friend. Be extremely honest; for example, "I'm having a problem and I really need some help." It is fine to want material things or health for yourself or loved ones, but first ask yourself what feeling would result from having the things for which you ask. I suggest praying for that feeling rather than the specific things.

GRATITUDE

Most religious traditions prescribe specific prayers or grace before meals as a means of thanking God for the food and for our physical sustenance. As with other spiritual practices, there is something to be gained from these rituals, or they wouldn't have survived for thousands of years. The more you can appreciate the spirit of the practice rather than merely following its form, the greater its value will be. Science is just beginning to appreciate the multifaceted benefits of spirituality.

Feelings of gratitude can elicit similar life-enhancing benefits. The most spiritual rabbi I have ever met suggests this ritual: As soon as you wake up each morning, even before getting out of bed, close your eyes and picture yourself in a scene that made you happy to be alive and for which you are still grateful to have experienced. You never would have had that experience if you weren't living, and you know that something equally wonderful can happen again. What a great way to instill an attitude of anticipation and appreciation for being alive.

Most of us tend to take life for granted. Suppose you choose instead to see your life as a gift, to be thankful for all that it has provided you—both the pleasure and the pain. Adversity can give you the opportunity for tremendous growth. You might not be too happy about it at the time, but in retrospect you can be grateful for the lessons you've learned.

Gratitude can produce powerful feelings of joy and self-acceptance. It is an attitude that anyone can choose to have, just as you can choose to be positive or negative, be forgiving or unforgiving, see the cup as half full or half empty. It has been my experience that when people choose to look at the up side of life, more positive things start to happen. It seems that we attract whatever feeling we radiate. When you focus on gratitude, wonderful things happen. When you focus on what you do have, not on what you don't have, you feel a sense of abundance, which enables you to let go of negative thoughts and attitudes.

This isn't easy to do. If you are feeling a great deal of fear and anger, it is especially difficult to superimpose gratitude, but if you can release some of those feelings through forgiveness and acceptance and put your heart into practicing gratitude, I know it will work for you.

As long as you are alive blessings will come your way. I rarely go through a day without thanking God for something, and every time I do there is an accompanying feeling of joy.

SPIRITUAL PRACTICES

Most major religions have their own variations on the following practices, but none of them needs to be performed in accordance with any particular ritual in order to be enjoyed. Doing them in whatever way is comfortable for you, or even creating your own ritual, will feel good. These basic practices involve fasting, the Sabbath, and the four fundamental elements of our world: earth, air, fire, and water.

Earth

Nature can give us a feeling of proximity to God and a healing energy that can't be found in most congested urban environments. I recommend spending as much time as possible outdoors in close contact with the earth, or at least in natural settings—parks, woods, beaches, or mountains. A daily walk is great, or playing a sport, riding your bike, swimming— especially in the ocean, a lake, or a river—gardening, or just finding a quiet or scenic spot to appreciate the surrounding beauty.

In 1981 Roger Ulrich, Ph.D., a professor of urban and regional planning at Texas A&M, performed a study with the help of Swedish scientists. He showed eighteen students slides of trees, plants, water, and cities. The students reported that the nature scenes, especially those of water, made them feel more elated and relaxed; in contrast, the urban scenes tended to elicit sadness and fear. Electroencephalograph (EEG) readings of the students' brain-wave activity showed significantly stronger alpha waves when viewing the nature scenes—scientific evidence of feelings of relaxed wakefulness.

In 1984 Dr. Ulrich found that exposure to nature speeds recovery from the stress of surgery. When he examined the hospital records of forty-six men and women who had undergone gallbladder operations, those with a window view of a small grove of trees were hospitalized about a day less than patients with a view of a brick wall. They also required less pain medication and were less upset.

Air

Find a place to meditate where the air is reasonably healthy. See the Meditation and Breath Therapy section in Chapter 12 for specifics on meditation.

Fire

Throughout the Bible, the dominant symbol for the divine essence in man is fire or light. Anyone who enjoys camping can attest to the pleasure of an open fire. A fireplace at home offers the same satisfaction, but because wood burning contributes to air pollution and sinus problems, I recommend a gas fireplace. The simplest and healthiest choice is to enjoy candlelight whenever possible.

Water

I have already emphasized the importance of drinking plenty of water. Now I am suggesting that you immerse yourself in it. There is nothing quite so relaxing as bathing in warm water. I suggest doing it at least once a day, morning or night. Hot tubs and spas are two of technology's greatest inventions, but if you don't have either, a bathtub will suffice. If you have ever soaked in a natural outdoor hot spring, congratulations—

you have experienced what I consider one of life's ultimate pleasures. Mineral hot springs can be therapeutic for a variety of ailments. In some that are unimproved (without a cement foundation), you can at times feel so close to nature that it is almost as if you are floating in the womb of Mother Earth.

Fasting   The ancient ritual of purification by abstaining from food can have a cleansing effect upon the body. According to the Bible, Moses and Jesus were both able to sustain fasts for forty days. Unless you have attained their level of spiritual mastery, please don't attempt a fast of that duration. I recommend one day, during which you abstain from both food and water. Doing this can definitely elicit a heightened spiritual feeling, as your focus shifts away from physical concerns. Select a day when work and family responsibilities are limited and you won't be too active. Plan for some quiet time alone, and during the final two hours of the fast drink six to eight glasses of water. This helps to cleanse your body of toxins. See how it feels after you have fasted once or twice, and if you think it has been beneficial, try fasting on a regular basis, perhaps monthly. You will be surprised at how much easier it is with each subsequent fast.

Sabbath

"Remember the Sabbath day to keep it holy." Although more than 3,000 years old, the Ten Commandments remain a worthy set of ethics. To the Jewish people, the Sabbath is still the holiest day on the calendar, even though it occurs every week. It is meant to be a day completely devoted to love—of God, self, family, and friends. I am not suggesting that you observe any particular day of the week or even a full day if you can't afford the time. For your spiritual health, however, I recommend setting aside the same time each week to indulge yourself in this celebration of life. Try to abstain from anything even remotely resembling work.

TOUCH

There are several topics that don't fit easily into one single component of holistic health but that offer several healing benefits simultaneously. Touch is one of them. I have included it here because it is not only one of our most effective healers, it might well be the most powerful and direct means of conveying love.

According to Saul Schanberg, M.D., Ph.D., a professor of pharmacology and biological psychiatry at Duke University, "Humans need to touch and be touched, just as we need food and water." His research and that of other experts on touch were cited in *Hands-on Healing*, edited by John Feltman.

- In a study involving forty premature infants, half of them were gently stroked for forty-five minutes a day; the other twenty were not. Although all were fed the same amount of calories, after ten days, the touched babies weighed in 47 percent heavier than the unstimulated group. The stroked babies were also more active, more alert, and more responsive to social stimulation.
- When a person's wrist is gently held by someone else, the heartbeat slows and blood pressure declines.
- Children and adolescents hospitalized for psychiatric problems show remarkable reductions in anxiety levels and positive changes in attitude when they receive a brief daily back rub.
- The arteries of rabbits fed a high-cholesterol diet and petted regularly had 60 percent less blockage than did the arteries of unpetted but similarly fed rabbits.
- Rats that were handled for fifteen minutes a day during the first three weeks of their lives showed dramatically less cell deterioration and memory loss as they grew old, compared with nonhandled rats.

Yet in spite of the many healthy reasons to touch and be touched by other human beings, Americans indulge very little in this simple pleasure. One study in the 1960s noted the number of touches exchanged by pairs of people sitting in coffee shops around the world. In San Juan, Puerto Rico, people touched 180 times an hour; in Paris, France, 110 times an hour; in Gainesville, Florida, 2 times an hour; and in London, England, the pairs never touched. The implications and possible causes of this phenomenon would entail a lengthy discussion, although I am sure the puritanical legacy of associating touch with sex has had a profound effect on American attitudes. William E. Whitehead, Ph.D., an associate professor of medical psychology at the Johns Hopkins University School of Medicine, believes that a significant part of the blame lies with the father of modern-day psychology, Sigmund Freud. "Freud encouraged austerity in dealing with children. And parents bought into that behavior," says Dr. Whitehead. People who aren't cuddled a lot as kids, he adds, tend to develop into nontouching adults. The cycle then repeats itself, generation after generation.

As an osteopathic physician, I learned very early in my medical training about the therapeutic value of the "laying on of hands." Although almost all of our courses and textbooks were the same as those used to train our allopathic (traditional) medical doctors, we were also taught a holistic approach to health care that included osteopathic manipulative therapy. Soft-tissue stretching (somewhat similar to massage) and adjustments or corrections in the position of the spine and other body parts (similar to chiropractic adjustments) are part of this therapy. It has taken me a while to realize that patients responded well to this treatment not only because of the prescribed techniques, but also because of the healing potential of the touch itself. I have learned since of other therapies in which touch is a primary healing ingredient. They are acupressure, the Alexander technique, applied kinesiology, Aston-patterning, the Berry method, chiropractic, craniosacral therapy, Esalen massage, the Feldenkrais method, Hellerwork, hydrotherapy, myotherapy, oriental massage, physiatry, physical therapy, polarity therapy, reflexology, Reichian therapy, Rolfing, sports massage, Swedish massage, therapeutic touch, and the Trager approach. I will not discuss the relative merits of these methods other than to say that all of them deserve to be recognized as legitimate disciplines in the full spectrum of the healing arts.

I have always viewed the practice of medicine as the business of caring. As our health care system continues to change radically, the most insidious shift has been the erosion of the doctor-patient relationship. As it becomes more impersonal, there is less mutual trust. Within the traditional medical community there is a greater fear of closeness, which leads to limiting the touching of patients to that which is strictly necessary in the course of a diagnostic evaluation. Sick people need the comfort of human touch more than healthy people—a reassuring pat on the shoulder, hand-holding, or even a hug. If caregivers are to do their best job, this powerful method of healing must be learned. Touch has to become a larger component of every physician's therapeutic black bag.

If you are interested in experiencing a hands-on healing technique, I suggest trying a practitioner of one of the many therapies previously mentioned. See how it feels and give it a fair trial. If it works for you, that's great. If it doesn't, try something else. In my experience two of these, acupressure and reflexology, have been effective in treating chronic sinusitis. They are described in chapter 15.

Touch is a gift you can give to yourself every day. It requires allowing yourself to receive and to feel deserving. If you are meditating, praying, or lying in the bathtub, try touching your chest over your heart in as gentle and compassionate a way as you know how. A loving touch is healing, no matter who gives it.

Animals are perfectly fine sources of tactile comfort, says Alan M. Beck, Sc.D., director of the Center for the Interaction of Animals and Society at the University of Pennsylvania. Numerous studies, he adds, "definitely show that petting an animal can lower one's blood pressure." Other doctors suggest that there are health benefits to be had even from cuddling inanimate objects—teddy bears, for instance. If you have neither a pet nor a favorite stuffed animal, my prescription for maintaining your spiritual health is to get several hugs daily!

There is no question that we have become too distant from one another. There is clearly a movement in this country to compensate for that deficiency and restore our sense of wholeness and balance. The trend toward more touching is a return to the norms and values of preindustrialized society. Primitive cultures are all very touch oriented. I have lived with one such native group in which touch is their primary method of healing. These people believe that their healers have a gift bestowed by God, and that the healing energy that flows through the healer to the patient is God's love. Whatever its source, the healers' touch works extremely well for a variety of ailments. By our standards these people might be considered primitive or underdeveloped, but they are clearly much healthier than most Americans in body, mind, and spirit.

SPIRITUAL HEALTH RECOMMENDATIONS: A SUMMARY

- Spirituality is *awareness of a power greater than yourself*, most commonly referred to as God. This divine power is the essence of all life on earth and is the spark or life energy within every human being.

- *Knowing or loving God and loving your neighbor as yourself* are the primary moral principles of most religions. As spiritual health objectives in contemporary American society, they can best be reached through first learning to love yourself. As you do, you will experience less fear in your life and a deeper sense of unconditional love for yourself and others. In that feeling lies a greater awareness of God.
- *Meaning, purpose, and intuition:* Begin by asking yourself what your life is about, where you're heading, and what you enjoy doing. This will help clarify your sense of purpose as well as provide the opportunity to give your gifts to others. Your intuition, or inner voice, is your best guide in the process. Take time to listen and be willing to risk in learning to trust it.
- *Prayer:* Daily prayers, those prescribed from your religious training or personalized "talking to God" prayers, are helpful. I also recommend Psalm 121 in the morning, Psalm 91 after work, and Psalm 23 before bed.
- *Gratitude:* Begin your day by visualizing a scene that makes you feel happy to be alive. Don't take life for granted; there are numerous blessings for which to be grateful. Focus on what you have, not on what you lack.
- *Spiritual practices:* Use the four basic elements of our world by engaging in outdoor activities that enhance closeness to the earth, meditating or using conscious breathing somewhere with clean air, using candles more often, and soaking daily in a warm bath, hot tub, or natural hot spring. Fasting for one day periodically and observing a regular weekly Sabbath (a day to focus on love, for yourself and others) are both effective practices.

- *Touch:* This is a basic human need that for most of us is filled far too seldom. There are many therapeutic disciplines in which touch is the primary attribute. If you are treating a chronic condition that has not responded to your present regimen, consider choosing one of these approaches. Remember, too, that hugs heal!

14 SOCIAL HEALTH

Social health comes from connections to other human beings. It requires the balance of autonomy with intimacy. I have found it to be the aspect of holistic health in which we Americans are most deficient, and it is clearly the most difficult for us to improve. The reasons for this social malaise will be a topic for much discussion in the coming decade. I have no doubt that it was aggravated by the self-involvement of the seventies and the compelling profit motive, greed, and win-at-all-costs attitude of the eighties expressed by the bumper sticker "He who dies with the most toys wins."

The origin of this social disease might be debatable, but its impact on the family—the very foundation of social stability—is unmistakable. As a society we are feeling the pain of a pervasive sense of isolation: a 50 percent divorce rate, a general sentiment of feeling overworked, dual-career marriages, and a generation of children more adrift and alone than any that has preceded them. According to *Turning Points*, the 1989 report of the Carnegie Council on Adolescent Development, almost half of all adolescents are at significant risk of reaching adulthood unable to meet the requirements of the workplace, to make the commitments to family and friends, and to accept the responsibilities inherent in a democratic society. They are susceptible to "a vortex of new risks . . . almost unknown to their parents and grandparents."

Our young people reflect the world we have shaped for them. What seems dysfunctional in teenagers' behavior actually might be functional ways of dealing with the crazy environment they have inherited. What they reflect is our lack of connectedness with others. This sense of alienation can create both social and physical disease. Dean Ornish, M.D., a professor at the University of California School of Medicine at San Francisco, found that the common denominator among heart disease patients was their feeling of hostility and a sense of isolation. The importance of social relationships can also be seen in the high incidence of illness and death after the loss of a loved one or even a simple move to a new city, state, or country. In a study conducted by Kenneth Pelletier, Ph.D., a professor of both medicine and psychiatry at the University of California School of Medicine at San Francisco, on terminal cancer patients with long-term survival, one of the strongest indicators was their relatively high degree of social involvement.

SUPPORT GROUPS

We humans are socially dependent animals, and the quality of our lives depends a great deal on our level of social integration. (A fascinating look at the human animal can be found in Desmond Morris's *The Naked Ape.*) Human babies have the longest infant dependency in the animal kingdom. A foal can run within hours of its birth; a kitten or puppy can leave its mother within two months. We humans are born helpless and stay dependent for years. If we don't bond and receive continual care, we die. Relatively little of our behavior is programmed at birth. Most of our learning, beliefs, attitudes, and worldview is shaped by an almost umbilical connection to our culture. The need to be a part of a social system does not diminish in adulthood; in fact, it becomes more elaborate. We look to society to provide food, shelter, goods, information, and health care. It is not surprising that we suffer when our link to others is broken. The recent scientific acknowledgment that support groups help people with chronic disease makes perfect sense. David Spiegel, M.D., conducted a study at Stanford University School of Medicine on women with metastatic breast cancer. All of the women received chemotherapy or radiation therapy. One half of them were in a support group that met weekly for one year. These women lived twice as long as those who were not in the support group. Whether a person has AIDS, multiple sclerosis, Parkinson's disease, or diabetes, there will be a support group available in most urban communities. Now sinus patients are joining these ranks. I have been meeting monthly with the SERI Sinus Sufferers Support System (S^5) at the Solar Energy Research Institute in Denver, the first sinus support group that has come to my attention.

There is a movement in America toward a greater sense of community. Small support groups for those sharing common values and goals are becoming much more commonplace. Men's groups, women's groups, and couples' groups, perhaps affiliated with a church or synagogue, are gathering all over the country, some for the purpose of enhancing spiritual growth, but all benefiting from the social connection. They meet regularly; some weekly, others twice a month, and some monthly. This is a positive and healthy indication of our nation's social recovery.

MARRIAGE

Marriage can be the most difficult, as well as the most rewarding, of all relationships. It can potentially become the most powerful spiritual practice in which we can engage. Most religions regard this bond between a man and a woman as a holy union. If humanity's fundamental moral principle is to "love thy neighbor as thyself," its practice begins not with the person living next door, but with the neighbor with whom we share our bed.

A healthy marriage incorporates all of the ingredients of holistic health, which is synonymous with learning to love. There is probably not a more effective vehicle for curing sinus disease than to work on your marriage or intimate relationship. The key to success is commitment to each other and to your growth, both that of the individual and that of the relationship. Once that pact is made, you will begin to recognize that the relationship is an entity that is greater than the two of you. As Maggie Scarf wrote in her book *Intimate Partners,* "When space is provided within the system—space for changing, growing, being different over the course of time—marriage can be the most therapeutic of relationships, the fertile terrain which permits both partners to expand, flourish, and attain their full potentials." Change entails letting go of parts of yourself, and as you do, you will realize that in giving more to the relationship you are ultimately giving to yourself.

Marriage also promotes physical health. People who are single, divorced, or widowed are twice as likely to die prematurely as those who are married. This is particularly true of men. In October 1990 a study at the University of California, San Francisco, found that single men between the ages of 55 and 64 are twice as likely to die within ten years as married men their age. For women, it is not marriage so much as having social support that lends a longevity edge. Unmarried people also wind up in the hospital for mental disorders five to ten times as frequently. So before deciding to divorce, you might want to ask yourselves if you have done all you could do to save the relationship.

After more than twenty-three years of marriage, my wife, Harriet, and I share with other couples what we have learned together. The recommendations that follow are distilled from the counseling the two of us have received; from our marriage counseling practice; from Harriet's master's-level education in social work and her certification in marriage and family counseling; from two insightful books, *Getting the Love You Want* by Harville Hendrix, Ph.D., and Maggie Scarf's *Intimate Partners*; and from our many years of working to make our own relationship a more conscious one. The following is a brief discussion of the methods and exercises we find helpful. If you are interested in making a deeper commitment to your relationship, I suggest you begin with marriage counseling. As with any new course of study, it doesn't hurt to find yourselves a good teacher.

Shared Vision

A vision is really a way of defining your mutual goals and focusing your energy on their attainment. Without a vision, your relationship can become directionless, and your problem-solving behavior will reflect a crisis orientation. You already might have completed your individual list of goals suggested in Chapter 11. Now each of you should write another in the form of affirmations in the present tense. These should be positive, short, descriptive, specific, and begin with "we." For example, "We trust each other," "We express our anger toward each other," or "We are very affectionate and touch each other daily." The shared list might include statements relating to the way you feel about each other, where you live, how you play together, how you resolve conflicts, what your sex life is like, and anything else that applies to your situation. After sharing your vision with your partner, combine the similar sentences on both lists to capture their essence and create a new composite list. Try to list the goals in the order of highest value. Each of you will rank them differently, so do the best you can. You might also note the ones that will be most difficult for you to fulfill. When you have completed this "mutual relationship vision," schedule a time every day to read it to each other, or record it on a cassette and listen to it together. Do this exercise daily for at least sixty days. This is just one of the sixteen exercises described in Dr. Hendrix's book. An accompanying workbook is available from his Institute for Relationship Therapy in New York City.

Listening Exercise

Most of us are very poor listeners. It amazes me at times how little we actually hear when we seem to be listening. Since communication is the foundation of any relationship, and listening is a critical aspect of effective communication, this exercise can go a long way toward creating greater intimacy.

Schedule an uninterrupted forty-minute block of time twice a week in a comfortable, relaxed, quiet setting. One person speaks for twenty minutes while the other listens without responding. Then the roles are reversed. The object is to be able to talk freely about whatever you're thinking or feeling without worrying about judgment or criticism. Under the usual circumstances, if we express something that makes our partner uncomfortable, we get a negative reaction right away. With this exercise the listener will still react to the words or ideas that trigger discomfort, but will not be allowed to respond. The more the listener focuses on his or her own reaction, the less he or she is actually listening. The more you practice listening, the better you become at letting go of your own thoughts and feelings and at focusing on those of your partner. Some people have described this exercise as almost meditative, as it requires you to empty your mind of your own thoughts as you listen.

As the speaker, try not to dwell on the relating of current events, but concentrate more on the feelings these situations have elicited in you. If you're the second speaker, avoid a critique of what your partner just said. In one version of this exercise, the couple is not allowed to comment on anything that was said during the exercise for up to three days following it.

For one of the two weekly sessions you might want to try doing it that way. It is definitely more of a challenge, but with even greater rewards. Creating a safe environment for expressing our feelings and allowing ourselves to be vulnerable with our spouses are extremely valuable tools for building trust, understanding, acceptance, and, at times, exhilarating feelings of intimacy. The last couple to whom we recommended this exercise said: "It felt wonderful to have his total attention," and "I really liked the fact that she was just listening without giving me any advice."

This exercise is described in more detail in Maggie Scarf's book *Intimate Partners*.

Requests

When you commit to each other, you enter into a relationship in which you have promised to give and receive love. Since each of us is different, what feels like love to one person might not even be noticed by another. Most of us attempt to love our partners in ways that feel like love to us, and are surprised when they do not react as we would. A good method of eliminating this problem is simply to tell each other what feels good. To ensure that you receive more of what you want, write three requests of your spouse. These should consist of actions or behaviors that you, the requester, perceive as most loving. Like the affirmations, the requests should contain only positive directions and should be as specific as possible. Some examples might be: I would like you to give me two hugs daily; I would like you to spend one afternoon each week with me; I would like you to buy me flowers once a week; I would like you to help me more with the cooking and cleaning. It can be quite a revelation when someone you have lived with for many years, a person whom you thought you knew well, tells you what they *really* need from you. This exercise helps explain your own feelings of betrayal when your loving actions were not reciprocated. We often expect our partners to be mind readers: "He should have known what I wanted"; "She ought to have been able to tell how I felt." We really can't know exactly unless we are told. Be specific, make requests, and get what you need. It is extremely important to thank your partner for complying with any request. This might not have been an easy or natural thing for him or her to do—otherwise you wouldn't have had to ask in the first place. Acknowledge the effort and even greater compliance might follow.

Having Fun Together

The pressures and responsibilities of daily life in America make it difficult to remember to have fun. For many couples, the glue that reinforces their relationship is the memory of enjoyment they shared during their courtship and early years together. To rekindle some of that earlier excitement and sweep away the cobwebs of routine and boredom, it helps to schedule fun activities together regularly. Plan a day or half-day each week to spend together away from home in an activity one of you has chosen. Alternate the responsibility for the choice of activity. Being out of the house, unaccompanied by friends or other family members, can help you focus attention on each other. Choosing something neither of you has ever tried before can add a sense of adventure to your play. If you can manage it, plan one weekend a month out of town. You might be surprised at how refreshing and invigorating regularly scheduled short trips can be for your relationship. These two-day excursions might be just what you need, especially if a real vacation isn't feasible.

PARENTING

Don't expect any quick fix or magic cures in this section. A magician I'm not—just another parent trying to do my best. I

have no simple approaches to what many see as life's most challenging full-time job. However, we can also choose to look at
parenting as one of life's most enriching experiences—as a
chance to play, to feel more in touch with our own "inner
child"—and to let go of ourselves and experience selflessness.
In dealing with teenagers, in particular, we are provided with
a wonderful vehicle for practicing forgiveness, unconditional
love, trust, self-acceptance, self-awareness, and most of all,
patience.

A useful guideline in the process of learning effective parenting might be to ask yourself regularly, "Will this (action,
response, activity, or demand) of mine help my child's self-
esteem?" The same principle holds true in parenting as it does
in marriage: *To love another is to help that person better love
himself or herself*. Obviously, as human beings, we are not always able to meet this ideal. Children are constantly trying to
expand their limits and are testing ours at the same time.
While they seek greater independence, our job is to balance
our own degree of comfort—which includes our values and
levels of fear, faith, and trust—with what will most benefit
these young explorers for whom we are responsible. It requires a great deal of awareness to appreciate who these
unique persons are and to know how best to provide them the
safety and base of security they need in order to develop their
independence and discover their hidden talents and gifts.
Most of us take great pride in our children's achievements and
strengths and disavow any connection to their flaws. Still, our
children are composites of genetic inheritance from both parents, environmental influences, and the intangible factor of
their own unique spirit. This combination produces a human
being altogether different from any other. As parents we must
respect and acknowledge this difference, even though at times
we feel as if our children are extensions of ourselves. What we
have considered to be good or bad for us might be just the opposite for our children.

In the field of family therapy, the family is usually seen from the "systems" approach. This view holds that if a member's behavior is harmful to himself or others, the problem and the solution lie not solely within that individual but in the entire family system. This perspective encourages parents to look at their roles and the partial responsibility they share for the problem. A child's crisis can be a mirror reflecting to a parent an imbalance in his or her own individual system as well as in the family system. One of the significant advantages of family therapy is that change often occurs more rapidly than in individual psychotherapy. In much the same way that holistic medicine refrains from treating the physical symptom without looking at the entire person, the systems approach recognizes the need for family therapy when one member of the family is suffering. If this is a situation that applies to your family, I strongly recommend family counseling.

I have mentioned that anger is a primary cause of sinus disease. The focus of that anger is often either yourself, your spouse, or your children. Now that you know several ways to release it, there is another way to use anger beneficially, particularly with regard to your children. I have found consistently that the aspects of a child's behavior that most upset a parent are those the parent likes least about him- or herself. I guess it's just easier to be angry with our kids than with ourselves. These disturbing behavior patterns become most apparent during adolescence, which merely adds to the challenge of parenting teenagers. For instance, suppose you believe your child has innate ability in a certain sport, with a musical instrument, or in a creative art, but the child refuses to pursue it for fear of making mistakes or looking awkward or silly as a beginner, or perhaps for no reason at all. You feel a very strong reaction, become furious, and find yourself insisting that the youngster at least *try* this new endeavor. Whenever you react so strongly, it's time to stop, reflect, and use the situation as a mirror. Perhaps this particular incident is reminiscent of your own fear of trying new things. It might be bringing up feelings of frustration and anger with yourself for the many times you failed to realize your own potential. Out of your anger with the child can arise a chance for you to see yourself more clearly and to forgive and accept both yourself and the child. Opportunities for loving often present themselves in unusual ways.

Good parenting requires both time and consistency. If you've completed a personal vision list and a shared vision list with your partner, they might provide a good idea of which values you would like to instill in your children. These values can serve as a guide for the rules you both implement and consistently adhere to as parents. Setting limits is just another way of loving your child and yourself.

Time seems to be the ingredient most lacking in today's society. In the typical American family both parents are employed outside the home, and the most striking change for this generation of teenagers is their isolation. A high percentage of these children have been with many different caretakers, often spending more hours with them than with their own parents. For these and many other reasons, this is not an easy period in which to be growing up in the United States. But even in the two-career household, if the commitment is there, time for the family can be found. Family dinners, for instance, when everyone eats together, don't have to be a lost tradition. I suggest trying to share at least this one daily meal as a chance to converse and get to know one another. Make sure the television is off. The average American watches about thirty hours of television a week, which must mean that it has become both a distraction from and a frequent guest at dinner tables across the country.

Other ways to spend time as a family are to worship together each week at church or synagogue and to designate a regularly scheduled time during the weekend for a fun activity. You can rotate the leader, so that each family member has a chance to choose the activity. The value of play cannot be overemphasized. Having fun together can sometimes accomplish what many sessions of family therapy are unable to do.

What parents really need to do is show that their love is unconditional, that nothing a child does or fails to do will diminish that love, and that children do not have the power to make or break their parents emotionally by their actions or achievements. That's really all there is to it! Isn't that simple?

ALTRUISM

The late Hans Selye, a pioneer in modern stress research, thought that by helping people you inspire their gratitude and affection, and that the warmth that results somehow protects you from stress. More recent studies suggest that this warm feeling might well come from endorphins—the brain's natural producers of euphoria. Even watching others help a third party seems to help the observer. In a striking study at Harvard University, psychologist David McClelland showed students a film of Mother Teresa, the embodiment of altruism, working among Calcutta's sick and poor. Analyses of the students' saliva revealed an increase in immunoglobulin A, an antibody that can combat respiratory infections. Even the students who consciously had no sympathy for Mother Teresa responded with enhanced immunity. Epidemiologist James House and his colleagues at the University of Michigan's Survey Research Center studied more than 2,700 men in Tecumseh, Michigan, for almost fourteen years to see how social relationships affected mortality rates. Those who did regular volunteer work had death rates two and one-half times lower than those who didn't.

The well-researched Type A personality—hard driving, hurried, and competitive—has a higher risk of heart disease than others. In a study performed by Duke University internist Redford Williams, M.D., it was found that the more hostile the person, the more his or her coronary arteries were blocked. At the University of Maryland, James Lynch, Ph.D., found that people who do not listen well, who jump at the first chance to answer back, tended to have higher blood pressure.

The evidence is mounting that selflessness not only feels good but is healthy. When we freely choose to care, we seem to get as much, or more, than we give. (However, as Ornstein and Sobel point out in *Healthy Pleasures*, being in control and having a choice are crucial to the health benefits of giving. Those who must care for sick loved ones for long periods often report more, not less, stress and illness.)

The closer our contact with those we help, the greater the benefits seem to be. By far my greatest rewards as a physician have come from the gratitude and appreciation I've felt from so many of my patients. Most of us need to feel that we matter to someone, but you needn't be in the healing arts to derive that pleasure. There is a growing number of needy people in our society—homeless, hungry, parentless, and illiterate— and there are many ways to help them.

The destructive self-centeredness underlying hostility can be treated with a healthy dose of selflessness. But the treatment works best if your generosity comes from the heart and is not calculated to benefit you. In *Healthy Pleasures*, Ornstein and Sobel devote a chapter to "selfless pleasures." They close with the following:

> Healthy altruism comes from the understanding that you and those around you are part of the same human community or social body. When one person suffers or is deprived, all of us are affected. It is for this reason that religions counsel generosity and service to others. The human community is strengthened and the server, too, benefits.
>
> It is important, even vital, to be able to connect with

other people and to be part of life in general; our lives, our health, and our destiny are connected with that of others. The great surprise of human evolution may be that the highest form of selfishness is selflessness.

SOCIAL HEALTH RECOMMENDATIONS: A SUMMARY

- Social health is defined by our degree of *connection to other human beings.* American culture has bred a society suffering from isolation, alienation, aloneness, and hostility.
- *Support groups* are small groups of people who meet regularly to share views on common ailments, problems, values, or beliefs, or for the purpose of enhancing spiritual growth. Anyone with a chronic disease or who feels a lack of community should consider either joining or forming a group.
- *Marriage* is a spiritual practice of learning to love your "neighbor" as yourself, balancing independence and intimacy. Some helpful exercises include sharing a vision listing common goals for the relationship; listening (one partner speaks for twenty minutes while the spouse listens without any response, then the reverse; requests make three requests of your spouse for actions or things that would make you feel loved; and having fun together regularly scheduling a block of time for enjoying each other's company.
- *Parenting* is a challenging opportunity to practice unconditional love on our children as well as ourselves. It requires a balance between teaching independence and allowing the exploration of potential gifts and setting comfortable limits. It takes consistency, time, and the recognition of your child's

uniqueness. Try to define your values and establish rules in accordance with them; create time for family dinners and family fun. Parenting might be life's most difficult and most rewarding full-time job.

- *Altruism*—helping others—can be pleasurable as well as providing a boost to the immune system. Healthy selflessness can be an antidote for the hostility underlying self-involvement. Helping others with genuine goodwill brings a powerful feeling of connection, a sense of unity, and the recognition that in giving to others you are ultimately giving to yourself.

15 A GUIDE TO HOLISTIC SPECIALTIES

What I have presented in chapters 7 through 14 is an introduction to and overview of holistic medicine. The material was meant to provide you with some idea of the breadth of this field and to give you enough information to begin to practice it on yourself. Conveying the full scope of this healing art would require an encyclopedic text.

As a general practitioner of holistic medicine, just as I did as a general practitioner of traditional medicine, I serve as a "jack of all trades," with a working knowledge of each component of holistic health. However, just as there are many medical specialties, there are also many holistic specialties. Most medical specialties focus on one part or system of the body; for example, ear, nose, and throat specialists work only on the neck and above, including the sinuses. Holistic specialties, on the other hand, might encompass all parts of the body but might be limited in the degree to which they address the various aspects of holistic health. Some holistic specialists focus solely on the physical, others on the mental or emotional. There are those who work almost exclusively on spiritual or social health. The common denominator in most of these healing arts and disciplines is that medical science has not recognized their validity, and therefore they have been largely ignored—in many cases even scorned—by many in the traditional medical community. In honoring its commitments to heal and to teach, holistic medicine involves an openness to complementary concepts as well as an understanding that what is not proven is not necessarily invalid.

The four holistic specialties that I will discuss briefly in this chapter are all physically oriented, although in theory they can treat body, mind, and spirit. They are naturopathic medicine, Oriental or Chinese medicine, homeopathic medicine, and reflexology. I have chosen these four because I have had personal experience with each one and know that all of them have been successful in treating chronic sinusitis.

NATUROPATHIC MEDICINE

Naturopathic physicians (N.D.'s) are specialists in natural medicine. They are trained at four-year naturopathic medical colleges and are educated in the conventional medical sciences. They treat both acute and chronic disease, and their treatments are drawn from clinical nutrition, herbal or botanical medicine, homeopathy, Oriental medicine, physical medicine, exercise therapy, counseling, acupuncture, and hydrotherapy. Some naturopaths might combine several or all of these therapies, whereas others might specialize in one specific area.

The basic principles of naturopathy are based on the concept that the body is a self-healing organism. The naturopathic physician enhances the body's own natural immune response through noninvasive measures and health promotion. Rather than treat the symptoms, naturopaths strive to uncover the underlying cause of patients' diseases, looking at physical, mental, and emotional factors. Health is seen not as the absence of symptoms, but as the absence of the causes of symptoms. Prevention and wellness are vital principles in naturopathy. These physicians are trained to know which patients they can treat safely and which ones they need to refer to other health care practitioners. As teachers, naturopaths facilitate the growth of patients' responsibility for their own health and spark the enthusiasm and motivation patients need to make fundamental lifestyle changes. The origins of naturopathic philosophy extend as far back as Hippocrates, who set forth the principles "Do no harm" and "Let your food be your medicine, and your medicine be your food."

As a distinct American health care profession, naturopathic medicine is almost 100 years old. Early in this century there were more than twenty naturopathic medical colleges. Today there are only two—in Portland, Oregon, and Seattle, Washington. In the 1940s and 1950s, with the advent of more technological medicine, the increased popularity of pharmaceutical drugs, and the belief that such drugs could eliminate all disease, naturopathy experienced a decline. During the past two decades, however, as more people have begun to seek alternatives to conventional medicine, it has seen a resurgence in popularity.

Naturopathy seems to be making its greatest contributions to the healing arts in the fields of immunology, clinical nutrition, and botanical medicine. Much of the vitamin and herbal regimen for the treatment of sinusitis and the strengthening of the immune system described in chapter 10 comes from naturopathic medicine.

CHINESE MEDICINE

Traditional Chinese medicine is the primary health care system currently used by approximately 30 percent of the world's population. It is believed to be one of the oldest medical systems in existence, dating back almost 5,000 years. The practice of acupuncture (a method of using fine needles to stimulate invisible lines of energy running beneath the surface of the skin) is the component of Chinese medicine most familiar to Americans, but the system also includes Chinese herbology, moxabustion (the burning of an herb at acupuncture points), massage, diet, exercise, and meditation.

In ancient China, doctors were not paid if patients under their care became sick. The job of the physician was to keep patients healthy. Chinese medicine believes that a certain process happens before the body develops a problem or disease. A Chinese medicine practitioner (O.M.D., Doctor of Oriental Medicine) looks for this process or pattern of disharmony. Through questioning, observation, and palpation, a practitioner can determine a person's current state of health and the problems that individual will be at highest risk for developing in the future. In this way, Chinese medicine is an effective preventive therapy.

Chinese medicine is based on a history, philosophy, and sociology very different from those of the West. Over thousands of years it has developed a unique understanding of how the body works. Practitioners of Chinese medicine see disease as an imbalance between the body's nutritive substances, called yin, and the functional activity of the body, called yang. This imbalance causes a disruption of the flow of vital energy that circulates through pathways in the body known as meridians. This vital energy, called qi or chi, keeps the blood circulating, warms the body, and fights disease. The intimate connection between the organ systems of the body and the meridians enables the practice of acupuncture to intercede and rebalance the body's energy through stimulation of specific points along the meridians.

People who have used Chinese medicine for a particular physical symptom frequently experience improvement in seemingly unrelated problems. This occurs because the Chinese approach tends to restore the body to a greater degree of balance, thereby enhancing its capacity for self-healing. The entire person is treated, not just the symptom, and the relationship of body, mind, emotions, spirit, and environment are all taken into account.

The World Health Organization has published a list of over fifty diseases successfully treated with acupuncture. Included on the list are sinusitis, asthma, arthritis, the common cold, headaches (including migraine), constipation, diarrhea, sciatica, and lower back pain. Acupuncture has also been effective in the treatment of allergies, addictions, insomnia, stress, depression, infertility, and menstrual problems.

Chinese herbs are the most common element of Chinese medicine as it is currently practiced in China. The herbs are becoming more popular in the United States, but it is still much easier to find a licensed acupuncturist (L.Ac.) than an O.M.D. who is knowledgeable about Chinese herbs as well as acupuncture. Pharmaceutical drugs are usually made by synthetically producing the active ingredient of an herb. Medicinal plants differ from the isolated active ingredients in synthetic drugs because they contain associate substances that balance the medicinal effects. Uncomfortable side effects are generally the result of the removal of these associate substances. Chinese herbs are capable of regenerating, vitalizing, and balancing the vital energy, tissue, and organs of the body without harmful side effects. They can be taken in pill or powder form or as raw herbs made into tea.

Chronic sinusitis can be treated effectively with a combination of acupuncture and Chinese herbs. I recommend seeing a licensed Chinese medicine practitioner who has a track record of success with herbs. Such practitioners are not that easy to find, but their numbers are increasing as more schools of traditional Chinese medicine are established in this country.

Acupressure works according to the same principle as acupuncture, using the same points on the meridians, but with direct finger pressure used in place of needles to stimulate these points. Of the two techniques, acupuncture is generally more effective, but acupressure allows you to do it yourself. The two diagrams in Figure 7 illustrate the acupressure points you can use for sinusitis. Pressure should be applied gently with your index fingers; abrupt application detracts from the relaxing effects. According to Cathryn Bauer in her book, *Acupressure for Everybody,* there are a few basic principles to keep in mind to know how to press points sensitively.

1. Your hands should be clean, warm, and dry. Start by holding your palm over the point for a moment. Then, using the tip of your index finger, probe the area gently until you feel a slight dip; this is the acupressure point.
2. Press in lightly, holding your finger in this position until you feel the muscle relax. Increase the pressure very slowly. Stop pressing when you feel that you're forcing it; just hold the pressure steady. Pay close attention to the way the point feels. Acupressure points often become warm as muscle tension eases.
3. Keep the pressure steady until the point is neither warm nor cool and pulses steadily. (The pulsation is not as strong as the pulse in your wrists and neck.) This usually takes at least three minutes, and it may take ten minutes or longer to release tensions if your symptoms are acute.
4. When the pulse is throbbing evenly, ease your fingertip off the point. An abrupt release can feel unpleasant.

Points 1, 2, and 3 are helpful for anyone with a sinus condition. Points 4 through 8 need only be used if those places are sore to the touch (using mild pressure). Stimulating these acupressure points can help to relieve sinus pain and congestion, as

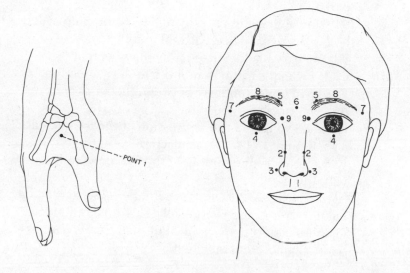

FIGURE 7   *Finger Acupressure*

well as the symptoms of nasal allergy. Keep in mind that symptom relief may not occur for up to thirty minutes. The points shown in Figure 7 are defined and described in the following material.

1. LI (large intestine) 4—in the webbing between thumb and index finger. To locate the exact point, place your thumb beside your index finger; the hump, or "meatiest" part, of the web is the spot. Stimulate both hands. This point addresses problems anywhere in your head, such as a headache, toothache, or eye or vision problem.

2. Extra bitong—along the edge of the nasal bone in the groove along the nose.
3. LI 20—beside the nose at the midpoint of its widest part.
4. ST (stomach) 2—in the tiny notch on the bony ridge below the eye, in line with the pupil.
5. UB (urinary bladder) 2—on the nasal end of the eyebrow in a small notch in the underlying bone.
6. Extra yin tang—midway between the nasal ends of the eyebrows.
7. Extra tai yang—in the depression of the temple (also a good point to use for headaches).
8. Extra yu yao—the middle of the eyebrow, in line with the pupil.
9. Along both sides of the bridge of the nose in the nasal corner of the eye socket. This is not an official Chinese acupressure point, but many sinus patients have obtained relief using it.

The Chinese herbs that are most effective for treating sinuses and are also used for allergies are Bi Yan Pian, Pe Min Kan Wan, Seven Forests-Xanthium 12, and Pollen Allergy.

HOMEOPATHIC MEDICINE

Homeopathy is a form of treatment that gently nudges the body toward a healthier state. Its practice was begun in 1820 by Samuel Hahnemann, a German physician, who believed that whatever caused disease would also cure it. The Latin phrase *similia similibus curantur* (like shall be cured by like) is the cornerstone of homeopathic medicine. According to Hahnemann, the proper remedy for an illness that exhibits any set of symptoms in a sick person is that substance that would produce the same set of symptoms in a healthy person.

This "law of similars" was not original with Hahnemann. The idea had been advanced by philosophers and physicians for thousands of years, and Hahnemann acknowledged his debt to Hippocrates, in whose writings the principle of "like cures like" appears. Hahnemann, however, was the first to build a consistent system based on this principle.

Homeopathy flourished in the 1800s and hasn't changed much since then. The Hahnemann School of Medicine in Philadelphia was originally a school of homeopathic medicine. The advent of rigorous scientific medicine in the United States during this century almost completely eliminated homeopathy. Today, this healing discipline is once again on the rise all over the world, including this country. The National Center for Homeopathic Medicine in Washington, D.C., estimates that there are somewhere between one and two thousand practitioners in the United States and that about 300 of them are M.D.'s or D.O.'s. Homeopathy has fared much better in other parts of the world. One-third of all French physicians practice it. In Britain, members of the royal family have been cared for by homeopathic physicians since the reign of Queen Victoria. Homeopathy is taught and used in hospitals and physicians' offices in Scotland, Germany, Austria, Switzerland, India, Mexico, Chile, Brazil, and Argentina.

Homeopathy uses infinitesimal or microdoses of natural materials—that is, mineral, plant, or animal. Some standard homeopathic solutions might be as weak as one part in a hundred thousand. These mixtures must be shaken vigorously (succussed) in a carefully prescribed manner in order to be activated. Only tiny amounts of a substance are used, but homeopaths believe that the treatment works because even if the substance were reduced to a single molecule, or lost altogether, its "pattern" would remain in the liquid and could produce an effect. Scientific support for this theory was contained in a 1988 issue of the prestigious British journal *Nature*. The publication described a study from a French laboratory headed by a well-known medical research scientist in the fields of allergy and immunology. The research team demonstrated that a solution that had contained a human antibody, yet was so diluted that not a molecule of it was left, had produced a response in human blood cells. Science cannot explain precisely how this could happen, but the reasons why many pharmaceutical drugs, including aspirin, are effective are also still largely a mystery.

Homeopathic medicines are not required to meet the safe and effective standards of the Food and Drug Administration. They are sold by mail, in drugstores, and in health-food stores. Most are nonprescription and legally can be advertised as remedies only for self-limiting conditions, such as colds. Prescription homeopathic substances can be dispensed only by someone licensed to prescribe drugs.

Most patients who seek the care of a homeopathic practitioner have a chronic condition considered incurable by traditional medicine. An effective homeopathic treatment for both acute and chronic sinusitis is kali bichromium at 30c every hour for four or five doses. I recently learned of a homeopathic nasal spray that works quite well. It is called Euphorbium Nasal Spray, which is manufactured in Germany and distributed by Biological Homeopathic Industries in Albuquerque, New Mexico.

REFLEXOLOGY

Reflexology is a science that makes use of the reflex areas in the feet and hands that correspond to all of the glands, organs, and parts of the body. It employs a unique method of using the thumb and fingers on the reflex areas to relieve stress and tension, improve blood supply and promote the unblocking of nerve impulses, and help the body achieve homeostasis—a state of balance. Reflexology is a natural, noninvasive therapy that grew out of the theories and techniques of acupuncture and acupressure. From hieroglyphic paintings found on a wall in an ancient Egyptian tomb, there is strong evidence to suggest that reflexology was practiced before 2330 B.C. From other ancient texts, illustrations, and artifacts, it is known that the early Japanese, Indians, and Russians, as well as the Chinese and Egyptians, worked on the feet to promote good health.

However, as with Chinese medicine, it was not until the twentieth century that reflexology gained acceptance in the Western world. Foot reflexology was introduced in the United States in 1913 by William H. Fitzgerald, M.D., following his discovery of the Chinese method of zone therapy. While serving as the head of the Nose and Throat Department of St. Francis Hospital in Hartford, Connecticut, he developed the modern zone theory of the human body, arguing that some parts of the body correspond to other parts and offering as proof the fact that applying pressure to one area anesthetizes a corresponding area.

In the 1930s, Eunice Ingham, a physiotherapist for Joseph S. Riley, M.D., another pioneer in the field of zone therapy, found the feet to be the most responsive areas for working the zones because they were extremely sensitive. Eventually she "mapped" all of the points on the feet that corresponded with points in other parts of the body. She discovered that an alternating pressure applied with the thumb and fingers on the various points on the feet had therapeutic effects far beyond the limited use to which zone therapy had been previously employed, including the reduction of pain. Thus, reflexology was born.

As with acupuncture, reflexology attempts to strengthen and balance the intangible life energy, chi or qi, that flows in zones or meridians throughout the body. Reflexologists specify ten energy zones that run the length of the body from head to toe—five on each side of the body ending in each foot and running down the arms into the tips of the fingers. Not only do these zones run lengthwise, but they pass through the body;

therefore, a zone located on the front of the body can also be reached from behind. All of the organs and parts of the body lie along one or more of these zones. Stimulating or working any zone in the foot by applying pressure with the thumbs and fingers affects the entire zone throughout the body. The actual physical mechanism that controls the ten zones in the body and feet is not fully understood, but it is a fact that reflexology is effective as an adjunct in the treatment of a variety of chronic ailments, probably as a result of its ability to induce deep states of relaxation. With this reduction of stress in the body, there are many potential benefits. Circulation can be improved, toxins and waste products can be eliminated more easily, energy levels can be increased, and mental alertness, creativity, and productivity can be heightened.

I can attest personally to the state of relaxation that results from a reflexology session, and I have known patients suffering from chronic sinusitis who experienced dramatic relief through this treatment. Reflex therapy can be administered through alternating finger pressure or percussion. This can be applied using the fingers (usually the index finger, with a rotating method of compression massage) and thumb, or using percussion machines. Under my desk, I keep a device called a Reflex-Aid, a floor-mounted foot massage machine equipped with a spiked rubber ball. This allows me to massage the foot reflexes while I'm working.

For anyone interested in trying this approach as a complement to their holistic health program, I recommend beginning with a visit to a reflexologist. See how it feels to have your feet worked on by a professional. Figure 8 illustrates the sinus points on the hands and the feet as well as the nose (allergies) and lung (bronchitis) points. Both hands have identical points in the webbing between the fingers. They can be stimulated with the thumb and index finger or even with the eraser of a pencil. Apply the pressure for twenty to thirty seconds and with enough force to cause some discomfort. The sinus points

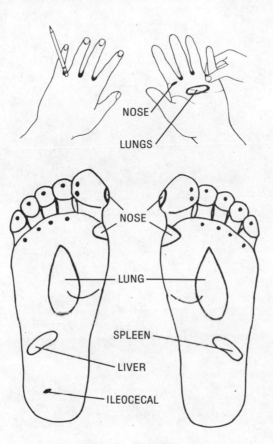

FIGURE 8   *Reflex Points*

are the same on the soles of both feet. There are also three other points—liver and ileocecal valve (both on the right foot) and spleen (on the left)—that are important in treating the sinuses. Try stimulating all of these points on a daily basis and see what happens. If nothing else, you will be giving your feet, one of our most abused body parts, some welcome attention.

16 MAKING IT HAPPEN

Having read this far in the book, you know now that the treatment of sinus disease can encompass the entire spectrum of medicine—from simply taking antibiotics to engaging in a process that might transform your life. If you choose, this transformation can help you make the transition from dependence on the medical profession to the recognition that you are capable of healing yourself. A human being, in fact, is an intrinsically self-healing organism, but we have developed many unhealthy habits that make it much more difficult for us to enjoy our lives fully.

In *Sinus Survival* I have shared with you my approach to health, derived from a healing odyssey that began with my roots in traditional allopathic medicine as the son of a radiologist, and that continued through the transitional stage of osteopathic medicine to my current work in what I believe will become the foundation of the health care system of the future: holistic medicine. What began as a desire to improve the condition of my sinuses has led me to a different style of medical practice, a cure for sinus disease and potentially any other chronic condition, and the recognition of a degree of personal health I had never imagined possible.

The only new aspect of this approach is that medical science is now, somewhat reluctantly, giving it a stamp of approval through the field of psychoneuroimmunology. Many so-called primitive cultures, much less technologically developed than our own, have instinctively practiced variations of holistic medicine. In the developed world holistic medicine is a comprehensive approach that incorporates everything from ancient healing practices to space-age technologies.

As a family doctor, I spent most of twenty years trying to find simple, quick, painless, and effortless remedies to satisfy my patients' requests for fast relief of their discomfort. During the past five years as a holistic physician, however, I've learned that a desire for the "quick fix" is one of the greatest obstacles to health. The approach I offer in this book synthesizes my family practice orientation as a "fixer" of symptoms, friend, and counselor (time permitting) with the focus of holistic medicine—the physician serving as a facilitator and teacher in the patient's own process of self-healing.

If you are willing to make the commitment to the holistic program, you will be giving yourself life's greatest gift. Its primary expense seems to be our society's most precious commodity: time. If you don't hurry, you've got it made, and you might be surprised to find that the program doesn't take nearly as much time out of your daily schedule as you thought it would. Many of the methods and practices I have described require only a heightened awareness on your part and no extra time. I highly recommend that you start by choosing only one or two methods in each component of health that require extra time. As you experience the rewards of practicing good health, you will be motivated to choose additional methods to expand your regimen. The following is a good example of how much time a beginning program might require. Every chronic sinus sufferer I have treated in the past five years has experienced either significant improvement or complete resolution of their condition within nine months of embarking on the sinus survival program.

PHYSICAL HEALTH

Eating and drinking are things you already do every day. Your new diet might entail no more than shopping for food at a different store and spending a bit more time initially on preparing some new dishes. Drinking more water and taking vitamins and herbs require awareness but negligible extra time. Aerobic exercise, at least three times a week for thirty minutes, is the major time consumer, but it's worth it. It may very well be the most valuable component of the entire program. Getting to and from, showering, and so on could make the actual time required for exercise closer to an hour. Averaged over a one-week period, including extra time for food shopping and cooking, physical health would require about **forty minutes** a day.

MENTAL HEALTH

Making a list of your goals, desires, and objectives for every realm of holistic health will definitely take some time, but the list serves as your guide for the rest of the program and has to be done only once. After rephrasing the goals into affirmations, reciting or listening to this list twice a day would probably require a total daily time of **five to ten minutes**. This could easily be done in the car or while commuting to and from work. Most of the other aspects of mental health—optimism, choice, humor, and forgiveness—entail only greater awareness, much of it derived from the daily recitation of the affirmations.

EMOTIONAL HEALTH

The primary objective of emotional health is to gain a greater awareness of your feelings. You can accomplish this to some extent just by identifying it as one of your goals. Meditation need take only five minutes twice a day. An anger-releasing technique—screaming, punching, stamping—can take just a minute or two. I recommend starting with these two methods. Regular participation in a sport or strenuous physical activity could doubly serve as aerobic exercise and a means of playing. The total daily time needed for emotional health is **ten to fifteen minutes.**

SPIRITUAL HEALTH

To gain a greater sense of God in your daily life, the only extra time initially needed might be to pray and recite psalms. This could take less than **five minutes** a day. Gratitude and listening to your intuition require only awareness and a conscious decision to slow down. Lighting candles takes little time, and if you meditate, pray, and recite affirmations while sitting in a hot bath you have created the perfect time-efficient holistic health treatment. Don't forget hugs, another all-purpose healthy quick fix.

SOCIAL HEALTH

The most valuable technique for feeling more connected to another person is the listening exercise. In the entire program, I'd rank it second only to aerobic exercise in its ability to profoundly change the way you feel in a short period of time. If you start with doing it once a week for forty minutes, that comes out to less than **six minutes** a day. Having family dinners requires no extra time and offers an excellent opportunity for relating to both your spouse and your children.

If you can make the commitment to give yourself just over an **hour a day** to practice good health, I can assure you it will make a profound difference in the quality of your life, not to mention how good your sinuses will feel. You will soon understand that health is much more than the absence of physical disease. As you gain a heightened awareness of the components of health, you will be more present with whatever it is you're doing; experience a greater level of physical fitness; let go of your ego and old, conditioned behavior patterns; take more risks; be more childlike and have more fun; be more accepting of pain; listen to your intuition and make better choices; spend more time with supportive people; be better able to give to others as well as to receive; see your life as a mirror reflecting back to you your unconscious thoughts and feelings; respect and better appreciate your home, the earth, and all of its inhabitants; trust and have more faith and much less fear; recognize that all of your dreams can become a reality and that anything is possible; and live while you're alive! This is holistic health.

BIBLIOGRAPHY

Adinoff, Allen D. "Difficult Asthma? Look for Sinusitis." *National Jewish Center for Immunology and Respiratory Medicine Medical Scientific Update*, February 1987.

Bandler, Richard. *Using Your Brain for a Change*. Moab, Utah: Real People Press, 1985.

Bauer, Cathryn. *Acupressure for Everybody*. New York: Henry Holt, 1991.

Carey, Benedict. "A Jog in the Smog." *Hippocrates*, May/June 1989.

Cherry, Rona. "The Best News of the Year." *Longevity*, May 1991.

Collins, John G. "Prevalence of Selected Chronic Conditions, United States, 1983–1985." National Center for Health Statistics: Advance Data, May 24, 1988.

Cooper, Robert K. *Health and Fitness Excellence*. New York: Houghton Mifflin, 1989.

Crowther, Richard L. *Indoor Air: Risks and Remedies*. Denver: Directions Publishing, 1989.

Feltman, John (ed.) *Hands-on Healing: Massage Remedies for Hundreds of Health Problems*. Emmaus, Pennsylvania: Rodale Press, 1989.

Gray, Henry. *Anatomy of the Human Body*. 8th ed., Charles Mayo Goss, ed., Philadelphia: Lea and Febiger, 1967.

Growald, Eileen Rockefeller, and Allan Luks. "The Healing Power of . . . Doing Good." *American Health*, March 1988.

Guyton, Arthur C. *Textbook of Medical Physiology*. Philadelphia: W. B. Saunders Company, 1968.

Hay, Louise L. *You Can Heal Your Life*. Santa Monica, California: Hay House, 1984.

Hendeles, Leslie, Miles Weinberger, and Lai Wong. "Medical Management of Noninfectious Rhinitis." *American Journal of Hospital Pharmacy*, November 1980.

Hendrix, Harville. *Getting the Love You Want: A Guide for Couples*. New York: Harper & Row, 1988.

Hersch, Patricia. "The Resounding Silence." *The Family Therapy Networker*, July/August 1990.

Joy, W. Brugh. *Joy's Way: A Map for the Transformational Journey.* Los Angeles: J. P. Tarcher, 1979.

Kozora, E. J. *American Holistic Medical Association's Nutritional Guidelines.* Seattle, Washington: American Holistic Medical Association, 1987.

Krakovitz, Rob. *High Energy: How to Overcome Fatigue and Maintain Your Peak Vitality.* New York: Ballantine Books, 1986.

Langs, Robert. "Understanding Your Dreams." *New Age Journal,* July/August 1988.

National Institute of Allergy and Infectious Diseases. "Sinusitis." Bethesda, Maryland, 1989.

Ophir, Dov, Yigal Elad, Zvi Dolev, and Carmi Geller-Bernstein. "Effects of Inhaled Humidified Warm Air on Nasal Patency and Nasal Symptoms in Allergy Rhinitis." *Annals of Allergy,* March 1988.

Ornstein, Robert, and David Sobel. *Healthy Pleasures.* New York: Addison-Wesley, 1989.

Patent, Arnold. *You Can Have It All.* Great Neck, New York: Money Mastery, 1984.

Peck, M. Scott. *The Road Less Traveled.* New York: Simon and Schuster, 1978.

Reid, Clyde. *Celebrate the Temporary.* New York: Harper & Row, 1972.

Siegel, Bernie S. *Love, Medicine and Miracles.* New York: Harper & Row, 1986.

South Coast Air Quality Management District. *Where Does It Hurt?: Answers to Questions about Smog and Health.* El Monte, California, 1988.

Togias, Alkis G. et al. Robert M. Nacierio, David Proud, "Nasal Challenge with Dry Cold Air in Release of Inflammatory Mediators: Possible Mast Cell Involvement." The American Society for Clinical Investigation, October 1985.

United States Environmental Protection Agency, Office of Air Quality Planning and Standards Technical Support Division. *National Air Quality and Emissions Trend Report, 1988.* Research Triangle Park, North Carolina, 1990.

Warga, Claire. "You Are What You Think." *Psychology Today,* September 1988.

INDEX

ABOUT THE AUTHOR

Dr. Robert S. Ivker completed his medical training in his hometown at the Philadelphia College of Osteopathic Medicine in 1972. In 1975, following a family practice residency at Mercy Medical Center in Denver, he opened a solo practice just outside the Mile-High City. The practice flourished and in 1983 he established Columbine Medical Center, currently a group of seven family physicians. He sold Columbine to Porter Memorial Hospital in 1986 and continued to work for another year as a family doctor and medical director of the center.

Since 1987, he has devoted his career to health education and the treatment of chronic disease, practicing holistic medicine, writing, consulting in environmental health, and public speaking.

Dr. Ivker has been board certified by the American Board of Family Practice, is a Fellow of the American Academy of Family Physicians, and is a member of the American Holistic Medical Association.

He lives with his wife, Harriet, and daughters Julie and Carin in Littleton, Colorado.

If you would like to know more about *Sinus Survival*; air; or if you have questions or information for Dr. Ivker, please write to Sinus Survival, P.O. Box 620236, Littleton, Colorado, 80162-0236.